The Role of AI, IoT and Blockchain in Mitigating the Impact of COVID-19

Edited by

S. Vijayalakshmi

Department of Data Science
CHRIST (Deemed to be University)
Pune Lavasa Campus - The Hub of Analytics
Maharashtra 412112, India

Naveen Chilamkurti

Department of Computer Science and Computer Engineering
La Trobe University, Melbourne
Australia

Savita

School of Engineering & Technology
Maharishi University of Information Technology Noida
Noida, Uttar Pradesh, India

Rajesh Kumar Dhanaraj

Symbiosis Institute of Computer Studies and Research (SICSR)
Symbiosis International (Deemed University)
Pune, India

&

Balamurugan Balusamy

Shiv Nadar University
Delhi-National Capital Region (NCR)
Greater Noida, Uttar Pradesh 201314
India

I0028957

The Role of AI, IoT and Blockchain in Mitigating the Impact of COVID-19

Editors: S. Vijayalakshmi, Naveen Chilamkurti, Savita, Rajesh Kumar Dhanaraj and Balamurugan Balusamy

ISBN (Online): 978-981-5080-65-0

ISBN (Print): 978-981-5080-66-7

ISBN (Paperback): 978-981-5080-67-4

need for a court order if at any point you breach any terms of this License Agreement. In no event will any delay or failure by Bentham Science Publishers in enforcing your compliance with this License Agreement constitute a waiver of any of its rights.

3. You acknowledge that you have read this License Agreement, and agree to be bound by its terms and conditions. To the extent that any other terms and conditions presented on any website of Bentham Science Publishers conflict with, or are inconsistent with, the terms and conditions set out in this License Agreement, you acknowledge that the terms and conditions set out in this License Agreement shall prevail.

Bentham Science Publishers Pte. Ltd.
80 Robinson Road #02-00
Singapore 068898
Singapore
Email: subscriptions@benthamscience.net

BENTHAM SCIENCE

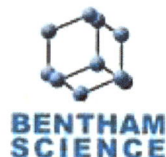

CONTENTS

PREFACE i

LIST OF CONTRIBUTORS ii

CHAPTER 1 ARTIFICIAL INTELLIGENCE (AI) IN BATTLE AGAINST COVID-19 1
Sivakumar Vengusamy and *Hegan A.L. Rajendran*
  INTRODUCTION 2
  AI-BASED TECHNIQUES IN THE BATTLE AGAINST COVID-19 3
      Particle Swarm Optimization (PSO) Technique 3
      Artificial Neural Network 4
      Model Estimation Procedures 4
      Random Forest 5
      Decision Tree 5
      Neural Network Models 6
  DATA PREPROCESSING FOR PRECAUTION MEASURES ON COVID-19 DATA 6
      Effective Measures on Datasets 7
          Weather Dataset 7
          Air Pollution Dataset 9
          Lockdown (Movement Restriction) Dataset 10
          Dataset Compilation 11
          Filtering of scope Dataset 11
          Drop Meaningless Variables 12
  TYPES OF MISSING VALUE IMPUTATION FOR AI MODELS 13
  OUTLIER TREATMENT FOR MACHINE LEARNING MODELS 15
  PREDICTIVE ANALYSIS: AI-MODEL CREATION 15
      Multiple Linear Regression 15
      Neural Network Regression 17
      Decision Tree 19
      Random Forest 21
  CONCLUSION 23
  ACKNOWLEDGEMENTS 24
  REFERENCES 24

CHAPTER 2 IMPACT OF 3D PRINTED COMPONENTS AND VENTILATORS ON COVID-19 26
K.T. Thomas, Lija Jacob and *Samiksha Shukla*
  INTRODUCTION TO CURRENT CORONAVIRUS DISEASE (COVID-19) 26
  THE UNPRECEDENTED SHORTAGE OF LIFE-SUPPORTING DEVICES AND VARIOUS COMPONENTS 27
  AN OVERVIEW OF 3D PRINTING / ADDITIVE MANUFACTURING 30
      Major 3-Dimensional Printing Technologies 33
          Binder Jetting 33
          Directed Energy Deposition 33
          Materials Extrusion 33
          Materials Jetting 34
          Powder Bed Fusion 34
          Sheet Lamination 35
          Vat Photopolymerization 36
      Common Additive Printing Materials 37
          Metals 37
          Polymers 37

     Ceramics 37

     Composite Materials 38

     Other Smart Materials 38

     Special Materials 38

   Application of 3D Printing in the Medical Industry/Healthcare Domain 38

     Preoperative Planning and Tailored Pre-surgical/Treatment 39

     Personalize Surgical Instruments and Prostheses 39

     Research on Osteoporotic Scenarios 39

     Enhancing Medical Practice 40

     Tissue Engineering 40

     Drugs that are Tailored to the Individual 40

THE ROLE OF 3D PRINTING, IN MANUFACTURING VENTILATOR COMPONENTS 40

THE ROLE OF 3D PRINTING IN MANUFACTURING COMPONENTS OF OTHER

MEDICAL DEVICES 43

   Face Masks 43

   Face Shields 44

   Nasal Swabs 44

   Other Potential Areas 45

CONCLUSION 45

REFERENCES 46

CHAPTER 3 IOT INNOVATION IN COVID-19 CRISIS 48

T. Genish and *S. Vijayalakshmi*

INTRODUCTION 48

IOT TECHNOLOGY IN COVID-19 49

   Perception Layer 50

   Network Layer 51

   Fog Layer 51

   Cloud Layer 52

APPLICATIONS OF IOT-ENABLED DEVICES 52

   Wearables 53

   Cardiovascular Monitoring 54

   Cardiovascular Sleep and Activity 54

   Respiration Monitoring 55

   Temperature Monitoring 55

ROLE OF DRONES TO COMBAT COVID-19 55

   Aerial Spraying and Monitoring of Crowds 56

   Cargo Delivery 57

   Temperature Scanning 58

     Lack of Understanding of the Use Case, Problem, and Scenario where Drones can

     add More Value During the COVID-19 Pandemic 59

     Lack of Support Systems 59

ROBOTIC TECHNOLOGY DURING PANDEMICS 59

   Growth of the Robotics Market 62

   Robotics After COVID-19 Pandemic 62

APPLICATIONS OF AI AND DIGITAL TECHNOLOGY IN COVID 19 63

   Healthcare 63

   Detecting COVID-19 Cases in Public Areas 64

   Contact Tracing 64

   Development of Drugs and Vaccines 66

CONCLUSION 67

ACKNOWLEDGEMENTS 67
REFERENCES 67

CHAPTER 4 POTENTIAL APPLICATIONS OF AI AND IOT COLLABORATIVE FRAMEWORK FOR HEALTH CARE 69
Lija Jacob, K.T. Thomas and Samiksha Shukla
INTRODUCTION 69
AI IN HEALTHCARE 71
    Early Detection of Disease 71
    Improved Decision Making 72
    Associated Care 72
    Easy Access to Healthcare Services 72
    End of Life Care 72
    Technology-Assisted Healthcare 73
    Challenges in AI and IoT Based Healthcare System 73
AI-IOT COLLABORATIVE FRAMEWORK 73
    Transformation of IoT with AI 75
    Benefits of AI-IoT Integration 75
    AI-IoT Convergence: Real-world Use Cases 76
    Autonomous Driving 76
    AI-driven Robots 77
    Embedding AI in Cybersecurity 77
    Artificial Intelligence (AI)-based Smart Appliances 77
        Smart Speakers 77
        Smart Laundry Machines 77
        Intelligent Refrigerators 78
AI-IOT CONTRIBUTION IN THE HEALTHCARE DOMAIN 78
    Patient Tracking and Predicting Staffing Requirements 79
    Diagnostics via Telemedicine or Remote Diagnosis 80
    Disease Management in Chronic Illness 81
    Addiction Management 82
        The Habit Tracker 82
        The AI-IoT Breath Analyzer 82
    Reduced Waiting Times in Emergency Rooms (ER); Fastest Attention to Critical Patients
    and Handling Shortages of Doctors 82
    Automated Robotic Processes 83
    AI-IoT for COVID-19 83
        Mass Screening in Pandemic 83
SMART HEALTH USING AI AND IOT 84
    Smartphone Applications Incorporating AI and IoT 85
        User Friendly 86
        Data Accuracy and Accessibility 86
        Easy Communication with Professionals 86
    Smart Wearables for Monitoring, Diagnosis, and Prediction 87
    AI-based Personal Emergency Response Systems (AI-PERS) 88
    Intelligent Drones 88
    Smart Kiosks 89
INTERNET OF MEDICAL THINGS (IOMT) FOR PANDEMIC OUTBREAKS 90
    On-Body Device Units 91
    In-home Segment 91
    Community Units 92

In Clinic Segment 92

Pros and Cons of IoMT 92

    Pros 93

    Cons 93

BLOCKCHAIN TWINNING WITH AI AND IOT IN HEALTHCARE 93

CONCLUDING REMARKS 94

ACKNOWLEDGEMENTS 95

REFERENCES 95

CHAPTER 5 ROLE OF SOCIAL MEDIA PLATFORMS TO MAINTAIN SOCIAL DISTANCING IN COVID-19 PANDEMIC 97

Sivakumar Vengusamy and *Danapriya Visvanathan*

INTRODUCTION 97

SOCIAL MEDIA AS DISEASE CONTROL IN TIMES OF PANDEMIC 99

TOP 3 REASONS FOR USING SOCIAL MEDIA PLATFORMS DURING THE PANDEMIC ...:. 100

    Seeking for Information 101

    Entertainment 102

    Shopping 103

DISCUSSION 103

    Importance of Social Media Platforms in Establishing As Well As Improving Social Distancing During the COVID-19 Crisis 103

        Spread of Information 104

        Creating Awareness 105

        Accurate Understanding 105

        Business Costs Saving 106

    Role of Social Media Platforms in Maintaining Social Distancing during the Pandemic 107

        A Source of Medical Information 107

        Social Media for Online Education 108

        A Marketing Platform 112

        Positive Thinking 113

    Impact of Coronavirus on the Use of Social Media 114

        The Social Media Participation 114

        The Social Media Demeanor 116

        The Online Shopping Journey 118

CONCLUDING REMARKS 119

ACKNOWLEDGEMENTS 119

REFERENCES 119

CHAPTER 6 AI BASED CLINICAL ANALYSIS OF COVID-19 INFECTED PATIENTS 123

Mohamed Yousuff, Rajasekhara Babu, R. Anusha and *M.A. Matheen*

INTRODUCTION 124

    Machine Learning (ML) 125

    Deep Learning (DL) 127

CLINICAL APPLICATIONS 130

    Treatment 130

    Diagnostics 131

        DL Models 132

        Diagnostics via Blood Tests 132

        Enhancing DNA Tests 133

    AI-based Mobile Applications 133

    COVID-19 Text Corpus Processing 134

Inspecting Infected Individuals 134
   Predicting Recovery and Mortality 134
   Predicting the Level of Disease Severity 135
   Monitoring Symptoms 136
COVID-19 EPIDEMIOLOGY 137
Pandemic Prediction 137
   ML-based Forecasting 137
   Clustering Strategies 139
   Neural Networks in Action 140
   Forecasting Regression Models 142
Containment of the Pandemic 144
   Evaluation of Risk 144
   Ensuring Safety Measures 144
   Combating False Information 147
Managing the Consequences 149
   Energy Services 149
   Assisting the Organizations 150
   Education and Sports 151
PHARMACEUTIC APPLICATIONS 152
Drug Repositioning 152
Immune System Analysis 154
Exploring the Molecular Structure of Medicine 155
Vaccine Development 155
UNDERSTANDING THE CONTAGION PATHOGEN 155
CONCLUSION 158
ACKNOWLEDGEMENTS 160
REFERENCES 160

**CHAPTER 7 CASE STUDY: IMPACT OF INDUSTRY 4.0 AND ITS IMPACT ON FIGHTING
COVID–19** 168
N. Hari Priya, S. Rajeswari and *R. Gunavathi*
INTRODUCTION 169
COVID-19 and Technology 170
CONCEPTUAL FRAMEWORK FOR INDUSTRY 4.0 170
Introduction 170
   I. Horizontal Integration Through Value Chains 171
   II. Vertical Integration and Networked Production or Service Systems 172
   III. End-to-End Value Chain Engineering 172
Key Characteristics of an Industry 4.0 System 172
Key Components 173
   Big Data Analytics 173
   Artificial Intelligence 173
   Internet of Things (IoT) 174
   Cloud Computing 174
   Cybersecurity 174
   Autonomous Robots 175
   Augmented Reality 175
BENEFITS OF ADOPTING INDUSTRY 4.0 175
Increase Efficiency 176
Collaborative Work and Enhanced Knowledge Sharing 177
Better Customer Experience 177

Reduces Costs 177
DESIGN PRINCIPLES 177
   Interoperability 178
   Virtualisation 178
   Decentralisation 178
   Real-Time Capability 179
   Service Orientation 179
   Modularity 179
ROLE OF INDUSTRY 4.0 IN FACILITATING THE PROMOTION OF SUSTAINABLE MANUFACTURING 180
   Sustainable Manufacturing 180
   The significance of Industry 4.0 technologies and their Benefits in Promoting the Sustainable Manufacturing 180
      I. IoT and IIoT 180
      II. Autonomous Robots and Cobots 181
      III. Virtualization 181
      IV. Additive Manufacturing 182
      V. System Integration 182
INDUSTRY 4.0 AND COVID–19 182
   What Effect did COVID-19 have on the Global Economy in 2020? 184
   The Impact of the COVID-19 epidemic in Daily Life 184
      A). Healthcare 185
      B). Economic 185
      C). Social 185
IMPACTS OF INDUSTRY 4.0 IN FIGHTING AGAINST THE COVID-19 186
   COVID-19's Effects on Mental Health 186
A STUDY ON THE MANUFACTURING INDUSTRIES 187
   Challenges Confronted by Manufacturing Industries in the Year 2020 188
ROLE OF DIGITAL MANUFACTURING IN THE COVID-19 ERA 189
OBJECTIVE OF THE STUDY 190
ANALYSIS AND FINDINGS 191
   Hindrances Faced Due to Work from Home Mode in Terms of Productivity 192
   Impacts Faced During COVID-19 192
   Lessons Learned from COVID-19 for Constructing the Production Process for the Future 193
      Make a plan to adapt to changing circumstances 193
      Demand Volatility can be Managed with On-demand Production 193
      Supply Chains Benefit from Mass Customizations 194
      A Worldwide Network Built on the Backbone of Regional Vendors 194
CONCLUSION 194
ACKNOWLEDGMENTS 195
REFERENCES 195

SUBJECT INDEX 199

PREFACE

Almost every country has been affected by the COVID-19 pandemic, which has had a significant impact on human lives and economic activity. The pandemic of COVID-19 was still significant in 2022, when millions of people around the world were getting sick. There has been an enormous and widespread impact on healthcare due to the COVID-19 pandemic; this has resulted in a significant and rapid increase in digital technology adoption. Luckily, digital technologies like Artificial Intelligence, the Internet of Things, and blockchain have unique characteristics such as immutability, decentralization, and transparency and can be used in many different fields like maintaining records, maintaining social distance, record maintenance, measuring mental health, and clinical analysis of infected people. Chap. 1 discusses artificial intelligence models in the battle against covid -19, with data preprocessing of three different datasets like weather dataset, air pollution dataset, and movement restriction dataset. Chap. 2 examines and describes how 3D printing technologies can be used as a weapon in the dangerous pandemic situation. Chap 3 discusses Iot, and Iot tools in preventing and controlling the virus. The chapter discusses several technologies that can be used in conjunction with IoT to combat the COVID-19 pandemic. The human society benefits from technologies during coronavirus outbreaks in terms of symptoms' diagnosis, contact tracing, quarantine monitoring, and social distancing. Numerous applications utilizing artificial intelligence in conjunction with the Internet of Things have been discussed. Chapter 4 illustrates the impact of artificial intelligence and the Internet of Things (IoT) in the healthcare domain, as well as the challenges that healthcare professionals face, particularly when dealing with a pandemic situation, and proposes some potential healthcare developments through the use of AI and IoT. The purpose of Chapter 5 is to raise awareness about the importance and role of social media platforms in preserving social distance between people. When discussing social media and the COVID-19 pandemic, there are usually three main points made: the importance of social media platforms in establishing and improving social distancing, the importance of social media platforms in maintaining social connections and interactions among individuals, and finally the impact of Coronavirus on social media use. Chapter 6 looks at AI techniques that are up to date in terms of COVID-19 in a number of different areas of interest. Treatment, diagnosis, prognosis of recovery, severity, and death of patients, chest X-Ray and CT-based analysis, pandemic prediction, control and management, pharmaceutical research and COVID-19 text corpus processing and virus detection are all performed with AI. A better understanding of various applications is needed to shed light on the current state of artificial intelligence in this pandemonium. Some suggestions and remarks about how to deal with the disaster are discussed in a better way. A better society can be achieved through the use of Industry 4.0 technologies and applications, which are explained in Chapter 7. Also, how Industry 4.0 contributes to sustainable manufacturing and the management strategies used to increase the company's efficiency, as well as COVID-19's impact are discussed.

S. Vijayalakshmi
Department of Data Science
CHRIST (Deemed to be University)
Pune Lavasa Campus - The Hub of Analytics
Maharashtra 412112
India

List of Contributors

Danapriya Visvanathan School of Computing and Technology, Asia Pacific University of Technology and Innovation, Kuala Lumpur, Malaysia

Hegan A.L. Rajendran School of Computing and Technology, Asia Pacific University of Technology and Innovation, Kuala Lumpur, Malaysia

K.T. Thomas Department of Data Science, CHRIST (Deemed to be University), Pune Lavasa Campus - The Hub of Analytics, Maharashtra 412112, India

Lija Jacob Department of Data Science, CHRIST (Deemed to be University), Pune Lavasa Campus - The Hub of Analytics, Maharashtra 412112, India

M.A. Matheen School of Computer Science and Engineering, Vellore Institute of Technology, Vellore, Tamil Nadu, India

Mohamed Yousuff School of Computer Science and Engineering, Vellore Institute of Technology, Vellore, Tamil Nadu, India

N. Hari Priya Sree Saraswathi Thyagaraja College, Pollachi, Tamil Nadu, India

R. Anusha School of Computer Science and Engineering, Vellore Institute of Technology, Vellore, Tamil Nadu, India

R. Gunavathi Department of Data Science, CHRIST (Deemed to be University), Pune Lavasa Campus - The Hub of Analytics, Maharashtra 412112, India

Rajasekhara Babu School of Computer Science and Engineering, Vellore Institute of Technology, Vellore, Tamil Nadu, India

S. Rajeswari Sree Saraswathi Thyagaraja College, Pollachi, Tamil Nadu, India

S. Vijayalakshmi Department of Data Science, CHRIST (Deemed to be University), Pune Lavasa Campus - The Hub of Analytics, Maharashtra 412112, India

Samiksha Shukla Department of Data Science, CHRIST (Deemed to be University), Pune Lavasa Campus - The Hub of Analytics, Maharashtra 412112, India

Sivakumar Vengusamy School of Computing and Technology, Asia Pacific University of Technology and Innovation, Kuala Lumpur, Malaysia

T. Genish KPR College of Arts, Science and Research, Coimbatore, India

CHAPTER 1

Artificial Intelligence (AI) in Battle Against COVID-19

Sivakumar Vengusamy[1,*] and **Hegan A.L. Rajendran**[1]

[1] *School of Computing and Technology, Asia Pacific University of Technology and Innovation, Kuala Lumpur, Malaysia*

Abstract: In Wuhan China, the world's most dangerous virus is discovered, which is named COVID-19 by World Health Organization. Social distancing is one of the powerful methods to control this virus as it is realized that lockdown is not a permanent solution. This research chapter aims to identify the major activities influencing the transmission of the coronavirus spread using Artificial Intelligence bound models. To conduct this research in the right direction, movement control restriction, meteorological parameters, and air pollution levels information are collected from various valid websites. End-to-end data pre-processing steps are carried out in detail to handle the outliers and missing values and investigate the correlation between dependent and independent variables. Multiple linear regression, neural networks, decision trees, and random forests are chosen to fulfil the objective of this research by identifying the most influential activities and other parameters. Here, the model's performance evaluation is done using the R^2 value, mean absolute error and mean squared error. The predicted values are plotted against the actual value to illustrate the error patterns. Among all models, random forest and decision tree models are proven to give the highest accuracy of 93 percent and 91 percent respectively. Prescriptive analysis has been further analyzed by performing feature importance extraction from the highly accurate models to identify the most impactful parameters the government authority and healthcare front-liners focus on to mitigate the number of COVID-19 cases daily.

Keywords: Artificial Intelligence, Coronavirus, COVID-19, Data Preprocessing, Dataset, Decision Tree, Feature Scaling, Linear Regression, Lock Down, Mean Absolute Error, Mean Square Error, Missing Value Imputation, Model Accuracy, Model Estimation, Model Performance, Neural Network, Outlier Treatment, Particle Swarm Optimization, Predictive Analytics, Random Forest.

---

* **Corresponding Author Sivakumar Vengusamy:** School of Computing and Technology, Asia Pacific University of Technology and Innovation, Kuala Lumpur, Malaysia, Tel: +91-9841253283, +91-9032874872; E-mail: dr.sivakumar@staffemail.apu.edu.my

---

S. Vijayalakshmi, Naveen Chilamkurti, Savita, Rajesh Kumar Dhanaraj and Balamurugan Balusamy (Eds.)
All rights reserved-© 2023 Bentham Science Publishers

INTRODUCTION

The world's most dangerous virus was discovered in late 2019 in Wuhan China, and was named COVID- 19 (SARS-COV2) by the World Health Organization, where 'CO' stands for corona and the 'VI' refers to the virus, and 'D' represents the disease. During this pandemic, veto-power countries like the United States and China accuse each other of spreading the virus. Many types of coronavirus present in the world can only cause mild sickness, but this COVID-19 is not like the previously identified virus [1].

The World Health Organization immediately decided to grab international attention by announcing this outbreak as a public health emergency. It is not a practical way for pharmaceutical companies to invent antiviral drugs right after a new virus is detected. So, the only option in politicians' hands to control the transmission is by implementing the movement restriction such as gathering cancellations, social distancing, sanitizing, corona patient contact tracking and isolation, non-essential business activities and the school shutdown, travel bans, and many more [2]. The intensity of movement restriction is based on the politician's decision and the seriousness of the corona cases in their country. The transmission of COVID-19 can be controlled during the initial stage of restriction, which shows a significant improvement.

However, the real problem only occurs when all business activities shut down, causing the country to hit an economic crisis due to an imbalance between the demand and supply of goods and services. This prolonged situation makes the country's financial sector unstable, leading to not having sufficient money to conduct research and development on vaccine creation, and the medical facilities in quarantine will be affected [3]. Even in the worst-case scenario, the country's economy needs to make money to keep the financial sector stable to retrieve the human community from a health crisis.

The coronavirus is known as a global crisis. Social distancing rules were recently introduced to the public to slow the spread of coronavirus cases, and the results show great improvement. However, the politicians and the business tycoons are not satisfied with the country's economy since most of the companies are shutting down and leading to the bankruptcy stage [4]. Even today, much research is involved in identifying the exact damage to the global economy due to this pandemic. The primary reason for the economic damage is the reduction in demand, which means there needs to be more customers to fulfill all the supplies of services and goods. For example, the restrictions to mitigate the news cases of COVID-19, especially in the tourism industry, were terribly affected, where the travelers could not buy flight tickets for their vacations or business trips. This issue forces the aviation industry to reduce the number of employees to cut operational costs. The same imbalance between supply and demand applies to almost all industries. Since the companies decided to lay off their employees to halt the revenue loss, the worry becomes worst among the unemployed who could not acquire the goods and services for their daily needs, and leads to a negative trend or impact on the economic graph. This indicates the clear damage, and the economist predicted that the value of gross domestic products globally would drop from 3°/c to 2.4°/c in 2020 [5].

Furthermore, the mortality rate due to coronavirus infection shows a significant spike in senior citizens with respiratory medical complications. So, air pollution is becoming a major factor in increasing the mortality rate because it affects the patients' willpower in their respiratory cycle. Moreover, certain meteorological conditions help the virus transmit easily through the air. Some proven researchers prove that the optimal temperature and humidity levels decrease the seriousness of coronavirus infections [6].

AI-BASED TECHNIQUES IN THE BATTLE AGAINST COVID-19

Since the outbreak has spread globally, AI approaches can help the medical community manage every step of the crisis and its aftermath, including detection, prevention, response, recovery, and research.

Particle Swarm Optimization (PSO) Technique

There are numerous studies being conducted on COVID-19 cases. The researchers are putting a lot of effort into innovating new techniques and utilizing several optimization techniques to safe humankind from this pandemic. Particle Swarm Optimization techniques are one of the well-known optimization approaches that Eberhart and Kennedy introduced in 1995. The idea of this technique is taken from the birds swarming and flocking behaviour [2]. In the real-time application, this procedure becomes eyes catching among the data scientists due to its simplicity. Other researchers have proved the particle swarm optimization on almost 28 different non-linear regression analyses. Moreover, the result indicates that more accurate results can be obtained with the minimum mean squared error (MSE) with fewer iterations. So, the regression analysis performance can be increased using the PSO techniques, and regression problems can be solved easily [7]. On the other hand, a comparison has also been made between the particle swarm optimization techniques and the statical techniques and it was concluded that the Mean Absolute Percentage Error (MAPE) is decreased by around 7 percent on the PSO than the ordinary statistical regression method. In the search space, the numerous swarms will be assigned with a certain velocity and the position where each swarm improved its position for the best within the search space given and uses the fitness model to conquer the best global position for the entire swarms' group.

Artificial Neural Network

Artificial Neural Network is the most famous prediction technique and was invented based on how the human brain's biological neuron works. To regenerate the biological neuron behavior, the artificial neural network contains some primary mathematical functions built on various building blocks called artificial neurons [8]. The data will be sent to an artificial neural network as an input, and then the built-in mathematical functions within the building blocks will produce the output. There are three basic principles in building the artificial neural network structure: the ANN architecture, mathematical functions and training algorithms. The ANN architecture can be divided into two main parts: single layer and multilayer. A single layer means the flow of information, and the neurons are organized in a layer while in the multilayer architecture, the information and the neurons are organized in multiple layers. The second phase is the training phase, which contains some mathematical functions to minimize the MAPE and MSE errors. The performance evaluation will be made based on the errors generated by the ANN, such as MSE, MAPE, RMSE and many more. Finally, the activation functions within the ANN will produce the output.

Model Estimation Procedures

Certain steps need to be followed to handle the complexities in the COVID-19 data, especially the meteorological datasets. First, the dataset needs to be handled carefully by studying the characteristics of the variables available with a descriptive statistical software. Then, without impacting any structural attributes, all the negative cells need to be eliminated with the data normalization techniques [9].

The next step is to identify the cross-section dependence in the data. If there are many global crises concurred, like the coronavirus pandemic, normally the data collected will face various issues in the statistical correlation during the model formation [10]. So, the data scientist needs to follow the rules on the cross-sectional dependence to be controlled. For the statistical interpretation, the stationary properties present in the dataset need to be assessed properly, and this can be done with the ClPS & CADF root techniques [11].

Finally, like cross-sectional dependence cooccurrences, the dataset might also undergo heteroskedasticity since time-series data are involved. [12] states that this issue can be solved easily by using the method called as Wald test for the group-wise regression model.

Random Forest

Breiman found an algorithm, which is known as a random forest, in the year 2001. He perfectly explained the techniques and approach of the algorithm's mechanism in his Springer book: "Machine Learning". He even compared all the techniques and mechanics with various learners. There are various advantages of Random Forest compared to other learners. Random Forest is one of the most well-predictive models, and the efficiency and effectiveness of prediction are known to be very high.

Especially in the healthcare industry, random forest algorithms are commonly utilized in DNA prediction DNA microarray data as the patient response is the tool used in Random Forest. Breiman (2001) [13] carried out an experiment in 2001, and they performed random forest prediction on the classification problem of different types of DNA microarray from various parts of the human's organs. Compared to other methods, Breiman (2001) concluded that Random Forest is a tough competition as it doesn't require the adjustment of parameters [13].

Various experiments have been performed that include gene expression profiles to show overall survival. The study is unique as it can help predict patient response using gene expression profiles. Their research shows numerous unique genes, around 100+ have been built using predictor methods like Nai've Bayes [14].

Decision Tree

Decision tree algorithms are most preferred among data scientists to build classification models in many domains. Several criteria have been used to select several essential attributes that have been constructed in the various level of trees. The invention is based on the splitting features, and they're also known as Gain Ratio, Average Gain and Gini index. There is another measurement called Average Gain as they use this measurement to overcome problems of Gain Ratio when it becomes zero, which leads to an undefined value [15]. The measurement is also a ratio between the number of unique attributes and Information gained. The new splitting method, also known as a distinct class-based splitting measure (DCSM) is proposed when the number of classes is considered. This measurement is divided into two different terms. Both products will decrease over time when the partition is considered pure. As a further process, the calculation will be made on the correlation ratio and the weightage of that specific features. The remaining feature will be updated from time to time -based on Correlation-Ratio [15]. This shows that this method provides way better accuracy than the available methods.

Neural Network Models

A neural network is the most well-known predictive model algorithm creation due to high accuracy chances during the prediction process. A neural network extracts valuable information and meaningful features from the original datasets. The most basic and intuitive neutral network is the fully connected one. It consists of a various number of neurons. Neurons collect input from other neurons, and non-linear transformations will be conducted that activate other hidden functions. Tentatively, a neural network can fit any intricate function that enables them to perform several tasks [16]. Yet, its performance and prices are opposite to each other. LSTM is a model that is used to predict time series data. The current output will be attached to the previous inputs to insert the neurons.

DATA PREPROCESSING FOR PRECAUTION MEASURES ON COVID-19 DATA

Data preprocessing needs to be handled carefully, and this stage consists of many processes and ¾ of the time in creating machine learning models will be spent here. The processes of data preprocessing is listed below:

• Univariate & Extended Data Dictionary Analysis

• Missing Value imputation

• Outlier Treatment

• Seasonality Analysis

• Bivariate & Correlation Analysis

Univariate analysis is the simplest form of analyzing data that covers central tendency (mean, median, mode) and dispersion (range, variance, quartiles, std deviation). The next step is the missing value imputation, where the null values will be identified. So, the null values can be replaced by mode or mean imputation. Since the dataset of this project is based on numeric values in all the variables, the mean imputation is the best approach to replace the null values. The outlier treatment will be done to improve the robustness of the model. Here, the distribution of the data points will be studied, and the gap between the mean and median or from the scatter plots will be calculated. If the gap range exceeds the tolerance level, then outliers are present in the dataset. These outliers can be eliminated by using the log transformation for the numeric values. Another sub-process of data preprocessing is seasonality analysis due to weather data and pollution levels involved in this project to study the seasonality pattern throughout the year [17]. Bivariate and correlation analysis studies the relationship between one variable and, or statistical measure, how two or more variables fluctuate together. The correlation can be divided into two categories: positive and negative. A positive correlation is when two or more variables are moving upwards or downwards parallelly, while a negative correlation exists when two variables are increasing or decreasing in the opposite direction. The correlation matrix will be used here to summarize the collinearity of all the variables available in the dataset.

Once the major step is done, the clean dataset must split into two different subsets with a ratio of 80:20. As a result, 80% of the observations will be used to train the model. The remaining 20% will be kept for verification. There are two machine learning models, which are unsupervised and supervised machine learning. Since the dataset contains the target variable, the supervised machine learning approach will take place to construct the model. Time series modelling, and multiple linear regression are the best options to understand the most influential factors towards the number of Corona patients.

Effective Measures on Datasets

Three different datasets are used in this study: Lockdown (Movement Restriction) Dataset, Weather Dataset and Air Pollution Dataset.

Weather Dataset

Since all three datasets are collected from various sources, the format of each dataset will not be in a standard structure. So, understanding the format and the structure is the most important to convert the format into a standardized one [18]. The weather dataset contains five columns with two values in each variable separated by delimiters. However, those two different values in each variable represent the same meaning with different conversions. The Fahrenheit unit in temperature variables will be deleted due to no significant difference to Celsius.

Text with Column

```
In [ ]: df_wea[['Avg_Temp', 'fre']]= df_wea['Temperature'].str.split('|', expand = True)
        df_wea[['Max_Temp', 'fre1']]= df_wea['Temperature max.'].str.split('|', expand = True)
        df_wea[['Min_Temp', 'fre2']]= df_wea['Temperature min.'].str.split('|', expand = True)
        df_wea[['Precipitation (mm)', 'Rainfall (inch.)']]= df_wea['Precipitation / Rainfall (mm) | (inch.)'].str.split('|', expand = True)

        # Dropping unwanted columns
        df_wea.drop(['Temperature, Temperature max.', 'Temperature min.', 'Precipitation / Rainfall (mm) | (inch.)','fre','fre1','fre2'], axis=1, Inplace = True)
```

```
In [ ]: df_wea
```

Out[7]:

	date	Avg_Temp	Max_Temp	Min_Temp	Precipitation (mm)	Rainfall (inch.)
0	Wednesday, January 1,2020	25°C	29°C	20°C	0.0 mm	0.0 inch
1	Thursday, January 2,2020	24°C	29°C	18°C	0.0 mm	0.0 inch
2	Friday, January 3,2020	25°C	31°C	19°C	0.0 mm	0.0 inch
3	Saturday, January 4,2020	25°C	31°C	19°C	0.0 mm	0.0 inch
4	Sunday, January 5,2020	25°C	31°C	20°C	0.0 mm	0.0 inch
...	...	...	...	...	...	...
361	Sunday, December 27,2020	25°C	32°C	19°C	0.0 mm	0.0 inch
362	Monday, December 28,2020	25°C	32°C	19°C	0.0 mm	0.0 inch
363	Tuesday, December 29,2020	25°C	32°C	19°C	0.0 mm	0.0 inch
364	Wednesday, December 30,2020	26°C	32°C	20°C	0.3 mm	0.0 inch
365	Thursday, December 31,2020	25°C	30°C	20°C	0.3 mm	0.0 inch

366 rows x 6 columns

Fig. (1). Deleting Duplicate Values.

After removing the unnecessary values (Fig. **1**) in the dataset, all the values in each variable show the unit of conversion description, such as '*C', 'inch' and 'mm'. These special characters need to be removed to make the observation readable by the machine as given in Fig (**2**). Another important point that needs to be realized is that initially, all the observations are along with strings which make the machine consider a string datatype in Fig. (**3**). These numeric observations will be converted into float datatype in Fig (**4**) except for the Date variable.

Remove Special Chars

```
In [8]: df_wea['Avg_Temp'] = df_wea['Avg_Temp'].str.replace(' oC','')
        df_wea['Max_Temp'] = df_wea['Max_Temp'].str.replace(' oC','')
        df_wea['Min_Temp'] = df_wea['Min_Temp'].str.replace(' oC','')
        df_wea['Precipitation (mm)'] = df_wea['Precipitation (mm)'].str.replace('mm',")
        df_wea["Rainfall (inch.)] = df_wea['Rainfall (inch.)'].str.replace('inch.','')
```

```
In [8]: df_wea
```

Out[9]:

	date	Avg_Temp	Max_Temp	Min_Temp	Precipitation (mm)	Rainfall (inch.)
0	Wednesday, January 1,2020	25	29	20	0.0	0.0
1	Thursday, January 2,2020	24	29	18	0.0	0.0
2	Friday, January 3,2020	25	30	19	0.0	0.0
3	Saturday, January 4,2020	25	31	19	0.0	0.0
4	Sunday, January 5,2020	25	31	20	0.0	0.0
...	...	...	...	...	...	...
361	Sunday, December 27,2020	25	32	19	0.0	0.0
362	Monday, December 28,2020	25	32	19	0.0	0.0
363	Tuesday, December 29,2020	25	32	19	0.0	0.0
364	Wednesday, December 30,2020	26	32	20	0.3	0.0
365	Thursday, December 31,2020	25	30	20	0.3	0.0

366 rows x 6 columns

Fig. (2). Removing Special Character.

Convert the numeric columns to FLOAT Weather

```
In [10]:   df_wea.dtypes

Out[10]:   date                     object
           Avg_Temp                 object
           Max_Temp                 object
           Min_Temp                 object
           Precipitation (mm)       object
           Rainfall (inch.)         object
           dtype: object
```

Fig. (3). Before the String Conversion.

```
In [11]:   df_wea.columns[1:]

Out[11]:   Index(['Avg Temp', 'Max_Temp', 'Min_Temp', 'Precipitation (mm)',
                  'Rainfall (inch.)'],
                 dtype='object')

In [12]:   for column in df_wea.columns[1:]:
               df_wea[column] = df_wea[column].astype(float)

In [13]:   # After
           df_wea.dtypes

Out[13]:   date                      object
           Avg_Temp                 float64
           Max_Temp                 float64
           Min_Temp                 float64
           Precipitation (mm)       float64
           Rainfall (inch.)         float64
           dtype: object
```

Fig. (4). After Conversion to Float Data Type.

Thus, the weather dataset is ready to be used for model creation.

Air Pollution Dataset

The air pollution dataset perfectly matches the weather data format where all the numeric values are known as floats except the Dale, and no special characters are involved. The air pollution dataset contains seven columns as given in Fig. (**5**) to show pollutant levels in the air. There are more than a year of observations present.

```
In [89]:   df_air
Out[89]:
```

	data	pm25	pm10	o3	no2	so2	co
0	Monday, February 1,2021	144.0000	123.0000	39.0000	17.0000	8.0000	13.0000
1	Tuesday, February 2,2021	130.0000	133.0000	39.0000	16.0000	12.0000	13.0000
2	Wednesday, February 3,2021	129.0000	130.0000	45.0000	19.0000	9.0000	13.0000
3	Thrusday, February 4,2021	145.0000	116.0000	40.0000	19.0000	7.0000	10.0000
4	Friday, February 5,2021	122.0000	196.0000	43.0000	21.0000	8.0000	9.0000
...							
424	Friday, January 3,2020	178.0000	195.0000	13.0000	24.0000	3.0000	10.0000
425	Thursday, January 2,2020	194.0000	128.0000	13.0000	24.0000	3.0000	10.0000
426	Wednesday, January 1,2020	188.0000	135.0000	11.0000	25.0000	3.0000	10.0000
427	Tuesday, December 31,2019	nan	140.0000	18.0000	22.0000	5.0000	10.0000
428	Monday, December 2,2019	nan	75.0000	9.0000	23.0000	1.0000	6.0000

429 rows x 7 columns

```
In [90]:  df_air.dtypes|

out[90]:  date     object
          pm25     float64
          pm10     float64
          o3       float64
          no2      float64
          so2      float64
          co       float64
          dtype: object
```

Fig. (5). Air Pollution Dataset Structure and Format.

Lockdown (Movement Restriction) Dataset

The movement restriction dataset is the core information for this project, indicating all the intensity levels of movement control order by the government. In this data, many unnecessary variables as shown in Fig. (**6**), such as currency, administrative levels, and coordinates are involved, which could be more useful for model creation. However, those variables are needed and can be used to fulfil the scope by filtering the Maharashtra state. There are better choices than deleting the process before combining all the datasets into one data frame.

```
In [92]:  df_lock.dtypes

Out[92]:  id                                         object
          date                                       object
          vaccines                                    int64
          tests                                       int64
          confirmed                                 float64
          recovered                                   int64
          deaths                                      int64
          hosp                                      float64
          vent                                        int64
          icu                                         int64
          population                                float64
          school_closing                              int64
          workplace_closing                           int64
          cancel_events                               int64
          gatherings_restrictions                     int64
          transport_closing                           int64
          stay_home_restrictions                      int64
          internal_movement_restrictions              int64
          international_movement_restrictions         int64
          information_campaigns                       int64
          testing_policy                              int64
          contact_tracing                             int64
          stringency_index                          float64
          iso_alpha_3                                object
          iso_alpha_2                                object
          iso_numeric                                 int64
          currency                                   object
          administrative_area_level                   int64
          administrative_area_level_1                object
          administrative_area_level_2                object
          administrative_area_level_3               float64
          latitude                                  float64
          longitude                                 float64
          Key                                        object
          key_google_mobility                        object
          key_apple_mobility                         object
          key_numeric                               float64
          key_alpha_2                                object
          dtype: object
```

Fig. (6). Movement Restriction Control Variables' Data Types.

Dataset Compilation

Three important parameters need to be specified in the merging process. Firstly, two different datasets need to be determined for the merging process and the common variable needs to be identified in both datasets, which will be used as a primary key. In addition, the type of merging method must be specified. Here, the primary key is 'Date', and the merging method is an inner joint. So, the common data in both datasets will be segregated in a single data frame.

Filtering of scope Dataset

The scope of this study is to provide a solution for the Maharashtra state, but the dataset contains information for all the states in India. Hence, Maharashtra state has figured out and formed a different data frame to fulfill the scope (Fig. **7**).

Filter Only Mumbai (Conditional Selection)

In [18] : df = df_com[df_com['administrative_area_level_2']== 'Maharashtra']

In [19] : df . to_csv("D:/Hegan's Project/Capstone/Dataset/Final.csv", index = False)

Fig. (7). Filtering the Scope.

Also, reverse cumulative calculation has been applied to identify the total number of corona patients each day. The number of confirmed cases on a particular date will be replaced with the difference from the previous date. This calculation also will be implemented on the recovered and deaths of corona patients.

In [122] : df . tail ( )

out [122] :

	id	date	vaccines	tests	confirmed	recovered	deaths	hosp	vent	icu	population	scho
293290	36222c2a	Sunday, December 27, 2020	0	0	1919550.0000	1809948	49254	0.0000	0	0	112374333.0000	
2994111	36222c2a	Monday, December 28, 2020	0	0	1922048.0000	1814449	49304	0.0000	0	0	112374333.0000	
294932	36222c2a	Tuesday, December 29, 2020	0	0	1925066.0000	1820021	49372	0.0000	0	0	112374333.0000	
295753	36222c2a	Wednesday, December 30, 2020	0	0	1928603.0000	1824934	49462	0.0000	0	0	112374333.0000	
296574	36222c2a	Thursday, December 31, 2020	0	0	1932112.0000	1828546	49520	0.0000	0	0	112374333.0000	

Fig. (8). Cumulative Number of Corona Patients.

Another issue formed by following this approach where the first row as 1st January 2020 data will subtract with the last day. Since the first corona patient was detected on 14th March 2020, the previous dates will all be considered 0 cases. So, the first-row data will be replaced with 0 cases. The complete process is shown in Fig. (8).

Drop Meaningless Variables

In a dataset, the chances of meaningless variables are very high, which need to be removed to advance its effectiveness and model efficiency. The meaningless variables can be identified by checking different types of observation in a particular variable. For example, a few variables are used to filter the location to be Maharashtra state, and this variable will only contain one type of data in all the rows. So, this kind of variable is considered meaningless and will not impact the machine learning models accuracy. There are several variables removed due to no meaningful data, which has been listed in the Fig. (**9**) below. After the removal of unwanted variables, the data frame consists of 27 variables with 362 observations.

Variables
id'
iso_numeric'
administrative_area_level_1'
administrative_area_level_3'
key'
key_numeric'
vaccines'
currency'
administrative_area_level_2'
latitude'
key_google_mobility'
key_alpha_2'
tests'
administrative_area_level'
longitude'
key_apple_mobility'
confirmed'
hosp'
recovered'
deaths'
vent'
icu'
population'
iso_alpha_3'
iso_alpha_2'

Fig. (9). Dropped Variables.

TYPES OF MISSING VALUE IMPUTATION FOR AI MODELS

The preprocessing steps are common and standardised for all the datasets, but certain aspects need to be improved: treatment, missing value imputation, skewness transformation and correlation analysis.

As stated in the figure below, the missing values are available in the 6 variables, mostly in the air pollution dataset.

Usually, there are numerous ways to replace or impute the missing values by mean imputation, mode imputation, forward-fill, backwards-fill, removing the whole observation, and many more. Since the null values are in the air pollution variables, replacing the values with the mean imputation method would provide an inconsistent pattern, and removing observation will affect the rule of thumb due to lack of observation [19].

The most appropriate way to find the possible values are forward-fill and backwards-fill or interpolation as computed in Fig. (**10**). In this research, the interpolation of missing value imputation has been applied to the dataset to find the average of the previous date and the following date data in Fig. (**11**). Accordingly, all the missing values have been replaced, and the data frame is free from null values.

```
Missing Values

Before Imputation

In [43]: df.isnull().sum()

Out[43]: date                                       0
         school_closing                             0
         workplace_closing                          0
         cancel_events                              0
         gatherings_restrictions                    0
         transport_closing                          0
         stay_home_restrictions                     0
         internal_movement_restrictions             0
         international_movement_restrictions        0
         information_campaigns                      0
         testing_policy                             0
         contact_tracing                            0
         stringency_Index                           0
         pm25                                      17
         pm10                                      19
         03                                         6
         no2                                       16
         go2                                       79
         co                                        50
         Avg_Temp                                   0
         Max_Temp                                   0
         Min_Temp                                   0
         Precipitation(nm)                          0
         Rainfall(inch.)                            0
         Rev_confirmed                              0
         Rev_recovered                              0
         Rev_deaths                                 0
         dtype: int64
```

Fig. (10). Missing Values Detection.

```
After Imputation

In [45]: df.isnull().sum()

Out [45]: date                                      0
          school_closing                            0
          workplace_closing                         0
          cancel_events                             0
          gatherings_restrictions                   0
          transport_closing                         0
          stay_home_restrictions                    0
          internal_movement_restrictions            0
          international_movement_restrictions        0
          information_campaigns                     0
          testing_policy                            0
          contact_tracing                           0
          stringency_index                          0
          p25                                       0
          pm10                                      0
          03                                        0
          ro2                                       0
          so2                                       0
          co                                        0
          Avg_Temp                                  0
          Max_Temp                                  0
          Min_TeMp                                  0
          Precipitation (mm)                        0
          Rainfall (inch.)                          0
          Rev_confirmed                             0
          Rev_recovered                             0
          Rev_deaths                                0
          dtype: int64
```

Fig. (11). Post Missing Value Imputation.

OUTLIER TREATMENT FOR MACHINE LEARNING MODELS

Outlier treatment is another vital step after missing value imputation. Outliers within the dataset are measured by calculating the distance of any observation that stays away from the rest of the data points cluster. Those detected outliers can be handled by two approaches: deleting observations and imputing observations. As the missing value section mentioned, deleting observations can be applied only when the dataset fulfills the rule of thumb requirements. Here, the outliers will be treated using the imputation method known as percentile outlier imputation. The outliers can be divided into two groups where extreme outliers are 3 times interquartile above 3rd quartile as an upper limit and 3 times interquartile below the 1st quartile as a lower limit. In contrast, while mild outliers can be considered as 1.5 times of interquartile range. However, in some cases, even though some data points are away from the determined quartile ranges, if there is no fault during the data entry process and those out-of-range data values are acceptable as truevalue and no further action is needed to treat them. First, the data points of each variable need to be visualized separately by using a boxplot to detect the variable which consists of outliers.

PREDICTIVE ANALYSIS: AI-MODEL CREATION

Multiple Linear Regression

Multiple linear regression is one of the most flexible algorithms in the data science world if the target variable in the dataset is numeric values. In this project, multiple linear regression was performed to build the predictive model using the sci-kit-learn library. The training dataset split of independent and dependent variables is inserted into the regression algorithms. After building the predictive model, the performance evaluation of the model will be determined with the help of the R^2 value.

The R^2 value is directly proportional to the accuracy of the predictive models, while the mean absolute error and the mean squared error are inversely proportional to the accuracy. So, during the testing process, the highest R^2 value with the lowest mean absolute error and the mean squared error model will be selected for the prediction.

Here, the R^2 value for the multiple linear regression is 0.72, which means 72 percent of accuracy can be provided during the prediction, as shown in Fig. (**12**). Moreover, the mean squared error and the mean absolute error for this model are 9229407.61 and 2281.27, respectively (Fig. **13**).

Evaluating the Model Performance

```
In [6]:  from sklearn.metrics import r2_score
         r2_score (y_test, y_pred)

Out[6]:  0.7172587129310771
```

Fig. (12). R² Value of Multiple Linear Regression.

```
In [10]:  mse_MLR = mean_squared_error (y_pred, y_test)
          mae_MLR = mean_absolute_error (y_pred, y_test)
          print ('Mean squared error using Multiple Linear Regression: ' , mse_MLR)
          print ('Mean absolute error using Multiple Linear Regression: ' , mae_MLR)

          Mean squared error using Multiple Linear Regression:  9229407.61987443
          Mean absolute error using Multiple Linear Regression:  2281.2703451651632
```

Fig. (13). MAE and MSE Value.

According to the results above, the accuracy of this multiple linear regression is 72 percent which is known as a poorly accurate model. In the healthcare industry, the accuracy should be more than 90 percent, and zero tolerance will be applied to those models which fall less than 90 percent. Based on the graph below, the data points of actual target variables have been plotted against the predicted target variable. As shown in the graph (Fig. **14**), the red line is known as the reference line of good prediction. If the predicted data points are close to the reference points, it shows the model with good prediction ability. However, the majority of the points are above the reference line, indicating that the model overpredicts the target variable.

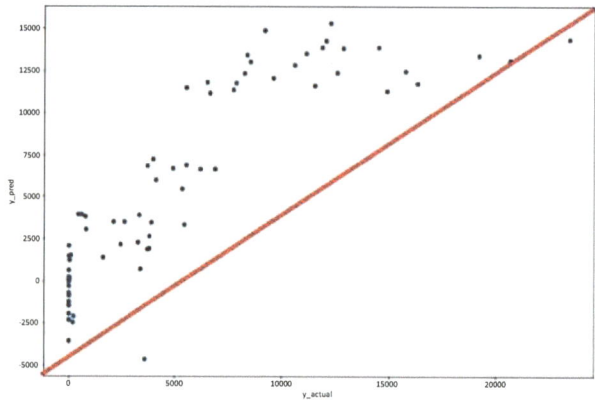

Fig. (14). Predicted Vs. Actual Values.

The Table **1** below shows the coefficient of the variables in the multiple linear regression where the intercept is stated in the first row. The difference between the prediction and the actual point is also listed.

Table 1. The Coefficient of the Variables.

Variables	Coefficient
Intercept	1.41654E+04
'school closing'	-1.56000E+03
'workplace closing'	-5.42000E+03
'cancel events'	5.16000E+03
'gatherings_retrictions'	-3.45000E+03
'transport closing'	-8.6lOOOE+O3
'stay home restrictions'	7.75000E+03
'internal_movement restrictions'	3.95000E+03
'international movement restrictions'	-2.17000E+03
'information_campaigns'	1.70000E+02
'testing_policy'	-1.09000E+03
'contact tracing'	1.70000E+02
'stringencyi ndex'	2.12000E+02
'pm25'	-2.19000E+00
'pm10'	4.10000E+01
'o3'	-1.59000E+02
'no2'	1.01000E+02
'so2'	7.09000E+01
'co'	-1.96000E+02
'Avg Temp'	-1.93000E+02
'Max Temp'	-5.85000E+02
'Man Temp'	4.27000E+02
'Precipitation (mm)'	-4.51000E+02
'Rainfall (inch.)'	7.41000E+03

Neural Network Regression

The neural network model has been utilized to predict the target variable for this project. To apply the neural network, the KerasRegressor library is used to perform the prediction since the target variables contain numeric values. To conduct the neural network, some basic settings must be applied in the KerasRegressor algorithms. Firstly, feature scaling should be done to ensure the observations are in the acceptable range. Feature scaling can be done in several ways, such as normalized scaler or standardized scaler.

Moreover, certain inputs need to be added in the algorithms to perform the prediction, such as the number of independent variables to be 23, the activation type is 'real', and the number of dense layers to be 2 as the first layer is 10240 while the second layer is 5120. The final output will be as 1 in the output layer.

After the training dataset is used to train the neural network model by settings 100 iterations, the neural network regression is ready for prediction. The prediction evaluation will be done exactly in Fig. (**15**) as the previous model with R^2, mean squared and mean absolute error. The R^2 value for the neural network regression is 88 percent and is considered more accurate than the multiple linear regression model (Fig. **16**). However, as mentioned earlier, zero tolerance will be applied especially, in the healthcare industry, and this model accuracy is considered prior since the cut-off point is 90 percent.

In [12]:
```
mse_MLR = mean_squared_error (predications, y_test)
mae_MLR = mean_absolute_error (predications, y_test)
print ('Mean squared error using NNR: ' , mse_MLR)
print ('Mean absolute error using NNR: ' , mae_MLR)
```

Mean squared error using NNR: 3806910.3138792906
Mean absolute error using NNR: 1129.5579075669916

Fig. (15). MAE & MSE Values for NN.

In [14] :
```
model.compile(loss="mean_squared_error", optimizer="adam", metrics=['nae'])
model.summary()
```

Model: "sequential _1"

Layer (type	Output Shape	persons #
dense_3 (Dense)	(None, 10240)	245760
dense_4 (Dense)	(None, 5120)	52433920
dense_5 (Dense)	(None, 1)	5121

Total persons: 52,684,801
Trainable persons: 52,684,801
Non-trainable persons: 0

In [15] :
```
history = model.fit(x_train_scaled, y_train, validation_split-0.2, epochs-100)
8/8 [--------------------------------------] - 2s 298vs/step - loss: 3071204:2500 - mae: 999:2950 - val_loss: 4451851-5000 - val_nae:
1357.4532
Epoch 82/100
8/8 [--------------------------------------] - 2s 293ms/step - loss: 3375775.2500 mae: 1063.6351 - val_loss: 4168772.5000 - val_ma
e: 1272.4073
Epoch 83/100
8/8 [--------------------------------------] - 2s 292vs/step - loss: 3131295.2500 mae: 993.2041 - val_loss: 4468811.0000 - val_mae:
1360.2380
Epoch 84/100
8/8 [--------------------------------------] - 2s 292ms/step - loss: 2824691.5000 - mae: 937.7085 - val_loss: 4320030.0000 val_mae:
1274.8378
Epoch 85/100
8/8 [--------------------------------------] - 2s 296ms/step - loss: 3153903.7500 - mae: 991.7751 - val loss: 4348999.0000 val_mae:
1323.9750
Epoch 86/100
8/8 [--------------------------------------] - 2s 295ms/step - loss: 3042564.2500 - mae: 962.8980 - val_loss: 4294688.0000 - val_mae:
1317.0948
Epoch 87/100
8/8 [--------------------------------------] - 2s 303ms/step - loss: 3045127.0000 - mae: 1009.2277 - val_loss: 4373281.0000 - val_ma
e: 1293.8973
```

Fig. (16). Training neural network regression model.

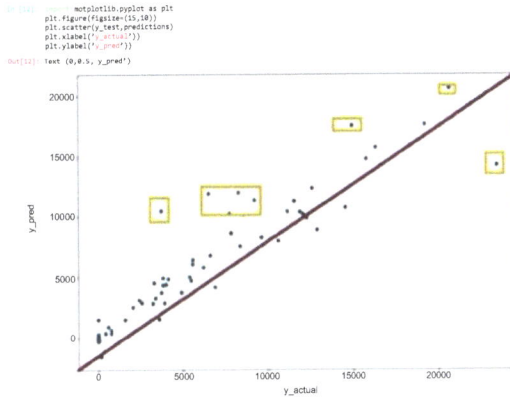

Fig. (17). Y Actual vs Y Predict values.

As per the Fig. (**17**), the red line is the reference line for good prediction, and the orange-coloured box is a misprediction value.

Decision Tree

A decision tree is one of the easiest algorithms to build predictive models. Here, the –sci-kit-learn DecisionTreeRegressor library has been used to form a model to predict the numeric target variables. The settings for the decision tree (Fig. **18**) are exactly the same as the multiple linear regression, where the training set of 80 percent will be used to train the model, and 20 percent of the testing dataset will be used for validation purposes.

Fig. (18). The Settings of the Decision Tree.

After training the predictive models, the performance evaluation shows the R^2 value of the decision tree is 91 percent accurate (Fig. **19**), which is an extremely good prediction model. The MSE and MAE values of the decision trees are 2824403.63 and 929.82 929.82, respectively (Fig. **20**).

Figs. (**21 & 22**) represent the Y actual *vs* Y prediction and the difference between Actual and Prediction of Decision Tree.

Evaluating the Model Performance

In [6]:   from sklearn . metrics import r2_score
r2_score(y_test, y_pred)

Out [6]:   0 . 913474889054647

Fig. (19). The R² value of Decision Tree.

In [10] :   mse_DCT = mean_squared_error(y_pred, y_test)
mse_DCT = mean_absolute_error(y_pred, y_test)
print('Mean squared error Using Decision Tree: ' , mse_DCT)
print('Mean absolute error Using Decision Tree: ' , mse_DCT)

Mean squared error Using Decision Tree: 2824403.6325506847
Mean absolute error Using Decision Tree: 929 . 8243835616437

Fig. (20). MAE & MSE values of Decision Tree.

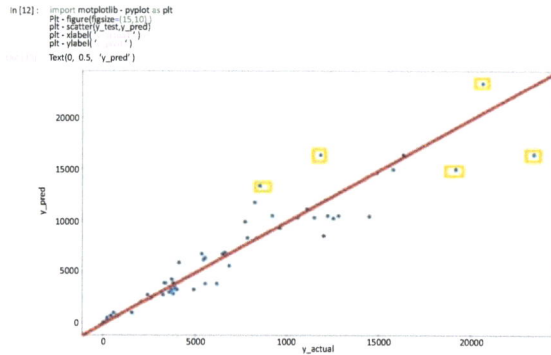

Fig. (21). Y actual vs Y prediction.

In [8] :   pred_y_df = pd . DataFrame ({ ' Actual ' : y_test, 'Predicted Value ' :y_pred, ' Difference ' :y_test - y_pred})

In [9] :   pred_y_df [0:20]

	Actual	Predicted Value	Difference
186	6603.0	6875.0	-272.0
274	12548.0	10244.0	-2304.0
45	0.0	0.0	0.0
26	0.0	0.0	0.0
217	12822.0	10483.0	2339.0
206	7717.0	9895.0	-2178.0
324	5439.0	6159.0	-720.0
158	3254.0	2739.0	515.0
113	778.0	728.0	50.0
6	0.0	0.0	0.0
170	3721.0	3214.0	507.0
159	3607.0	3007.0	600.0
191	6497.0	6741.0	-244.0
60	0.0	0.0	0.0
133	1606.0	1026.0	580.0
136	2078.0	2091.0	-13.0
306	6870.0	5585.0	1285.0
296	5363.0	6738.0	-1375.0
190	7827.0	8308.0	-481.0
145	2598.0	2436.0	162.0

Fig. (22). Difference between Actual and Prediction of Decision Tree.

Random Forest

The extended version of the decision tree is Random Forest. The steps for setting up AI algorithms are almost similar. The random forest repressor library will be applied, as shown in the Fig. (**23**). In this algorithm, 150 estimators have been set for the prediction models.

Training the Random Forest Regression model on the whole dataset

```
In [4]:  from sklearn . ensemble import RandomForestRegressor
         regressor = RandomForestRegressor(n_estimators = 150, random_state = 0)
         regressor . fit(x_train, y_train)

         RandomForestRegressor(n_estimators=150, random_state=0)
```

Predicting the Test set results

```
In [5]:  y_pred = regressor . predict(x_ test)
         np . set_printoptions (precision=2)
         #print(np.concatenate( (y_pred. reshape(len(y_pred),1), y_test.reshape(len(y_test),1)),1))
```

Fig. (23).   Training the Random Forest.

The R^2 value of this random forest predictive model is 93 percent (Fig. **24**) which is the best among the rest because the highest accuracy is achieved among all other models. Besides that, the mean squared and absolute error are 2279606 and 881, respectively (Fig. **25**). The error scores are maintained as low as possible to reach the most accurate model as shown in Figs. (**26 & 27**).

Evaluating the Model Performance

```
In [6] :  from sklearn.metrics import r2_score
          r2_score(y_test, y_pred)

Out[6] :  0.9301646407646629
```

Fig. (24). R^2 Value of Random Forest.

```
In [10] :  mse_RF  = mean_squared_error( y_pred, y_ test )
           mae_RF = mean_absolute_error(y_pred, y_test )
           print( "Mean squared error Using Random Forest:" , mse_RF )
           print( "Mean absolute error Using Random Forest:" , mse_RF )

           Mean squared error using Random Forest:  2279606 . 927396393
           Mean absolute error Using Random Forest:  881 . 0774986301369
```

Fig. (25).   MAE & MSE Value of Random Forest.

In [8]: pred_y_df =pd. DataFrame({'Actual' : y_test ,'Predicted Value': y_pred, 'Difference' : y_test-y_pred})

In [9]: pred_y_df [0:20]

out [9]:

	Actual	Predicted value	Difference
186	6603.0	6192.880000	410.120000
274	12548.0	12134.520000	413.480000
45	0.0	0.093333	-0.093333
26	0.0	0.613333	-0.613333
217	12822.0	10205.053333	2616.946667
206	7717.0	11430.840000	-3713.840000
324	5439.0	5228.993333	210.006667
158	3254.0	3041.753333	212.246667
113	778.0	604.006667	173.993333
6	0.0	0.000000	0.000000
170	3721.0	3333.540000	387.460000
159	3607.0	3442.520000	164.480000
191	6497.0	9303.653333	-2806.653333
60	0.0	0.000000	0.000000
133	1606.0	5172.797267	-3566.797267
136	2078.0	2241.920000	-163.920000
306	6870.0	4542.033333	2327.966667
296	5363.0	5606.326667	-243.326667
190	7827.0	9124.620000	-1297.620000
145	2598.0	2288.306667	309.693333

Fig. (26). The Difference Between Actual and Prediction.

In [12]: import matplotlib.pyplot as plt
plt.figures(figsize = (15,10))
plt.scatter(y_test,y_pred)
plt.xlabel('y_actual')
plt.ylabel('y_pred')

Out [12]: Text(0, 0.5, 'y_pred')

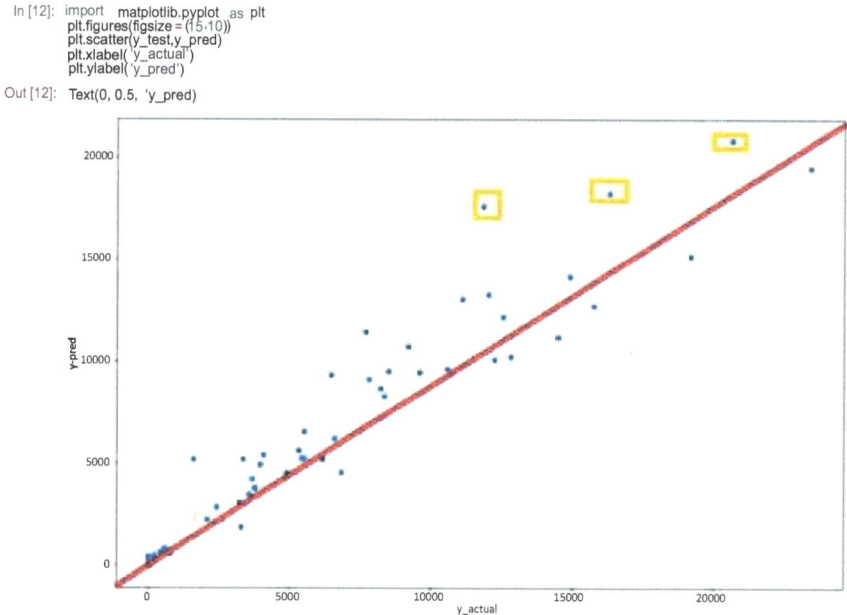

Fig. (27). Y Actual *vs* Y Prediction.

All four models' accuracy and error values have been listed in the Table **2** for comparison purposes. Among these four machine learning models, the decision tree and the random forest value of R^2 are 91 percent and 93, percent respectively.

Those two predictive models are good machine learning models for prediction since they fall above the cut-off level. Furthermore, the MAE and MSE scores of these two models are maintained at the lowest possible compared to the multiple linear regression and the neural network regression.

Table 2. Machine Learning Model Accuracy Comparison.

	MLR	**NNR**	**DCT**	**RF**
R-Squared	0.717258713	0.883375969	0.913474889	0.930164641
MAE	2281.270345	1129.557908	929.8243836	881.0774986
MSE	9229407.62	3806910.314	2824403.633	2279606.927

So, the best models chosen to conduct further analysis are the decision tree and the random forest.

CONCLUSION

The two most accurate predictive models have been provided with the most influential parameters contributing to the coronavirus transmission rate. The top 15 most influential parameters in movement control, meteorological, and air pollution levels have been highlighted in descending order. The random forest model suggests that O3, precipitation, stringency index, testing policy, pm25, internal movement restriction, gathering restrictions, pm10, transport closing, NO2, minimum temperature, maximum temperature, and rainfall must be kept in control to break the transmission of coronavirus. According to the decision tree model, the predictive model suggests similar parameters as a random forest except for the workplace closing. Even in the decision tree model, the gap between the workplace closing and the rainfall is huge, and this can be considered as not a highly impactful restriction.

Moreover, government authority needs to pay more attention to or take action in reducing air pollution levels where the air pollution parameters have a huge impact on the transmission of the virus. If the air pollution is controlled, the rainfall, precipitation and the surrounding temperature will automatically change accordingly. These air pollution issues will affect not only the corona patients but the overall healthy lifestyle of the residents. Furthermore, international movement restriction is one of the best ways of restricting the foreign virus into the country and encouraging people to refrain from using public transport in this critical situation. Gathering restrictions need to be enforced to maintain social distancing.

The internal movement restriction, stay-home restriction, school closing, workplace closing, contact tracing, information campaigns, and cancel events do not provide little contribution towards the number of new Corona patients. Hence, these types of activities can continue without any further restriction, but certain precautions must be taken to protect themselves from being infected. By implementing this, at least the student's education will not be affected, and the economy of the country can be recovered by avoiding workplace closing.

Even though these models were produced with high accuracy, there are still certain returns that can be improvised for data collection accuracy where the gathering restriction is implemented in Mumbai city, but the social distancing cannot be obeyed in such a compact area, and it's known as impossible to them. The COVID-19 testing tool is quite expensive for those people who are living in the slums, and they cannot be able to afford the testing tool. The accuracy of the data collection of a number of new cases might be faulty.

Based on this study, the government authority and the front-liners from the healthcare industry can take these two models as a reference to mitigating the number of coronavirus cases but can only be implemented in a real-world situation by testing in a real situation. Precautions are always the best option to stay safe from the dangerous virus.

ACKNOWLEDGEMENTS

All authors contributed to the study conception, design, and material preparation. Hegan A/L Rajendran performed data collection and analysis. The draft of the manuscript was written by Sivakumar Vengusamy, and he wrote all the versions of the manuscript. All authors read and approved the final manuscript.

REFERENCES

[1]   R. Eberhart, and J. Kennedy, *A new optimizer using particle swarm theory.* 1995.
[http://dx.doi.org/10.1109/MHS.1995.494215]

[2]   M.A. Behrang, E. Assareh, A.R. Noghrehabadi, and A. Ghanbarzadeh, "New sunshine-based models for predicting global solar radiation using pso (particle swarm optimization) technique", *Energy,* vol. 36, no. 5, pp. 3036-3049, 2011.
[http://dx.doi.org/10.1016/j.energy.2011.02.048]

[3]   Y. Chang, R.J. Huang, X. Ge, X. Huang, j. Hu, Y. Duan, Z. Zou, X. Liu, and M.F. Lehmann, "Puzzling haze events in china during the coronavirus (COVID-19) shutdown", *Geophys. Res. Lett.,* vol. 47, no. 12, p. GL088533, 2020.
[http://dx.doi.org/10.1029/2020GL088533] [PMID: 32836517]

[4]   M. Marvi, and A. Arfeen, "Demystifying a hidden trend: do temperature variations affect COVID-19 virus spread?", *SSRN Electr 1,* p. 3567084.
[http://dx.doi.org/10.2139/ssrn.3567084]

[5]   Y Wu, W Jing, J Liu, Q Ma, J Yuan, Y Wang, M Du, and M. Liu, "Effects of temperature and humidity on the daily new cases and new deaths of COVID-19 in 166 countries", *Sci Total Environ..*

2020, 729: 139051.
[http://dx.doi.org/10.1016/j.scitotenv.2020.139051]

[6]   R. Xu, H. Rahmandad, M. Gupta, C. DiGennaro, N. Ghaffarzadegan, and M.S. Jalali, "Weather conditions and COV lD-19 transmission: estimate and projections", *SSRN Electr 1*. 2020.
[http://dx.doi.org/10.1101/2020.05.05.20092627]

[7]   E Conticini, B Frediani, and D. Caro, "Can atmospheric pollution be considered a co-factor in extremely high level of SARS-CoV -2 lethality in Northern Italy?", *Environ Pollut*, vol. 261, p. 114465, 2020.
[http://dx.doi.org/10.1016/j.envpol.2020.114465]

[8]   R.R. Dangi, and M. George, "Temperature, population and longitudinal analysis to predict potential spread for COV lD-19", *SSRN*, 2020.
[http://dx.doi.org/10.2139/ssrn.3560786]

[9]   S.A. Sarkodie, and P.A. Owusu, "Global assessment of environment, health and economic impact of the novel coronavirus (COVID- 19)", *Environ. Dev. Sustain.*, 2020.
[PMID: 32837273]

[10]   "vantarakis. a cl, apostolou t. COVID-19 and Enviromental factors. A PRISM A-compliant systematic review"", *medRxiv*. 2020.

[11]   M. Eberhardt, and F. Teal, "Econometrics for grumblers: a new look at the literature on cross- country growth empirics", *J. Econ. Surv.*, vol. 25, no. 1, pp. 109-155, 2011.
[http://dx.doi.org/10.1111/j.1467-6419.2010.00624.x]

[12]   W. Grant, H. Lahore, S. McDonnell, C. Baggerly, c. French, J. Aliano, and H. Bhattoa, "Evidence that vitamin D supplementation could reduce risk of influenza and COVID- 19 infections and deaths", *Nutrients*, vol. 12, no. 4, p. 988, 2020.
[http://dx.doi.org/10.3390/nu12040988] [PMID: 32252338]

[13]   L. Breiman, "Random forests", *Mach. Learn.*, vol. 45, no. 1, pp. 5-32, 2001.
[http://dx.doi.org/10.1023/A:1010933404324]

[14]   T.M. Khoshgoftaar, M. Golawala, and J. Van Hulse, "An empirical study of learning from imbalanced data using random forest", *IEEE International Conference on Tools with Artificial Intelligence*, pp. 310-317 2007.
[http://dx.doi.org/10.1109/ICTAI.2007.46]

[15]   R. Changala, A. Gummadi, G. Yedukondalu, and U.N.P.G. Raju, "Classification by decision tree induction algorithm to learn decision trees from the class-labeled training tuples", *International Journal of Advanced Research in Computer Science and Sofiware Engineering, Vol*, no. 2, pp. 427-434, 2012.

[16]   S.F. Ardabili, A. Mosavi, P. Ghamisi, and F. Ferdinand, "V arkonyi -kciczy ar, reuter u, rabczuk t, atkinson pm, "covid- 19 outbreak prediction with machine learning", *SSRN*, p. 35501, 2020.

[17]   H. Li, X.L. Xu, D.W. Dai, Z.Y. Huang, z. Ma, and Y.J. Guan, "Air pollution and temperature are associated with increased COVID-19 incidence: A time series study", *Int. J. Infect. Dis.*, vol. 97, pp. 278-282, 2020.
[http://dx.doi.org/10.1016/j.ijid.2020.05.076] [PMID: 32502664]

[18]   N. Scafetta, "Distribution of the SARS-CoV-2 Pandemic and Its Monthly Forecast Based on Seasonal Climate Patterns", *Int. J. Environ. Res. Public Health*, vol. 17, no. 10, p. 3493, 2020.
[http://dx.doi.org/10.3390/ijerph17103493] [PMID: 32429517]

[19]   M. Travaglio, Y. Yu, R. Popovic, L. Selley, n.s. Leal, and L.M. Martins, "Links between air pollution and COVID-19 in england", *Environ Pollut.*, vol. 268, p. 115859, 2021.
[http://dx.doi.org/10.1101/2020.04.16.20067405]

CHAPTER 2

Impact of 3D Printed Components and Ventilators on COVID-19

K.T. Thomas[1,*], Lija Jacob[1] and **Samiksha Shukla[1]**

[1] *Department of Data Science, CHRIST (Deemed to be University), Pune Lavasa Campus - The Hub of Analytics, Maharashtra 412112, India*

Abstract: The disease caused by a virus known as the novel Coronavirus, also known as "COVID-19" by the public, was classified as a major epidemic by the World Health Organisation in 2019. Each country across the globe is affected by COVID-19. While writing this, over 150 million people were affected by the fast-spreading deadly pandemic, and over 3.5 million deaths due to COVID-19 were reported worldwide as per WHO's official COVID-19 dash panel-https://covid19.who.int/Economy and social life of no territory on earth was left unaffected by the COVID-19. Now vaccines are ready, it may take a reasonable amount of time to complete the vaccination process. One major challenge was the need for more support equipment like Beds, Oxygen Cylinders, and Ventilators. Improvisation in the mass production of many critical components, especially those supporting 3D printing technology, has shown some well-managed results in handling the shortage of many critical components. This chapter examines and describes how 3D printing technologies were used during the dangerous pandemic. It aims to describe many 3D-printed devices like face masks, face shields, various valves, *etc*. It also makes an effort to point out the dominant drawbacks of additive manufacturing technology in this area and examines the options for a future pandemic.

Keywords: 3D printing, Additive Manufacturing, Additive Printing Materials, Assistive respiration, Berating machine, Coronavirus, COVID-19, Extrusion based 3D printing, Lamination based 3D printing, Life-supporting devices, Lung disease, Materials Jetting, Pandemic, Photo Polymerization 3D printing, Powder-based 3D printing, Pulmonary infections, Shortage of ventilators, Ventilator components, Ventilator valves, Ventilators.

INTRODUCTION TO CURRENT CORONAVIRUS DISEASE (COVID-19)

Coronavirus Disease 2019, also known as COVID-19, was declared a pandemic by the World Health Organisation in 2019. So far, it has claimed the lives of peo-

* **Corresponding Author K.T. Thomas:** Department of Data Science, CHRIST (Deemed to be University), Pune Lavasa Campus - The Hub of Analytics, Maharashtra 412112, India; E-mail: thomas.kt@christuniversity.in

S. Vijayalakshmi, Naveen Chilamkurti, Savita, Rajesh Kumar Dhanaraj and Balamurugan Balusamy (Eds.)

ple from nearly every country on the planet. Over 150 million people were infected with COVID-19, and 3.5 million died as a result of the virus, although the figure is likely to be higher because many people died from complications after treatments, even if the virus was negative after treatment.

This pandemic was lethal and affected almost every corner of the world. The economy and social life of people changed and even destroyed. Though vaccines are now ready and all the countries are vaccinating their citizens, we can simply understand that it may take more months to complete the vaccination process. Many countries are yet to start vaccinating citizens under 18 years of age. Safe vaccination for children is still under trial. Lockdowns and other restrictions are still there in place. Many countries still insist on travel restrictions for different countries, and even restricted movement between states. The health departments are working day and night to control the pandemic. Mass production of many weapons like masks, sanitizers and other personal protective kits started in many countries, and now are adequate. However, now the globe is facing another problem, the unavailability of enough support equipment like beds, oxygen cylinders, and ventilators. Oxygen cylinders and ventilators were extremely required because most deaths were due to multi-organ failure, which was the effect of severe pulmonary infections. All medicines other than preventive vaccines have been made available till now.

Recent studies reveal the presence of a delta variant of Coronavirus which is more harmful and may affect the children critically and cause a fast blowout in schools when unvaccinated faculty members and other staff have close indoor proximity to the children. It should be noted that the majority of the children have not yet been vaccinated, and they have had indoor contact with unvaccinated children. Even though children are less affected than adults, they can get sick and spread it to adults who come into contact with them. Making the children obey the social distancing rules in schools is challenging. These facts show that COVID-19 will stay with us on the globe for at least several months. Proper support is needed for the people suffering from COVID-19. Governments are supposed to support healthcare workers by making available the required equipment to combat the pandemic.

THE UNPRECEDENTED SHORTAGE OF LIFE-SUPPORTING DEVICES AND VARIOUS COMPONENTS

The novel Coronavirus enters into our body mainly through the droplets from an affected person when they cough or sneeze, or at times, these droplets may be released from the mouth when a person talks. The virus thus moves down the affected person's respiratory tract. The respiratory tract includes the lungs.

Several researchers have been focusing on a protein known as the angiotensin-converting enzyme 2 (ACE2) "receptor," which allows the coronavirus to latch on to and attack many types of cells in the human body. There is high chance that COVID-19 can travel deeper than other viruses that cause the commonly known cold because it has more ACE2 receptors in the lower airway. This condition may lead to pneumonia, which is actually due to the contamination of the alveoli (miniature air balloons) present in the human lungs. It is in these tiny air sacs where the blood exchanges carbon dioxide and oxygen [1].

Most patients who lost their lives due to COVID-19 were hit hard with lung infections by the novel Coronavirus. A critical issue in the respiratory system of humans appears to be the reason for vulnerability to mortality in case of many people who were identified with COVID-19. Lungs of the patients were observed with diffuse alveolar damage and capillary fibrin thrombi. A study by Roden *et al.* (2019) reveals that acute bronchopneumonia and aspiration pneumonia also cause death in COVID-19-affected cases.

Acute lung injury seems to be the most difficult condition of SARS-CoV-2 infection, and the resulting related disorders, coronavirus disease 2019 (COVID-19), which causes pulmonary damage and even death in some people [2].

In most cases where severe lung problems occur, and breathing becomes difficult, medical practitioners recommended using a mechanical ventilator.

A ventilator is a mechanical device that helps a person to breathe in case they have difficulty breathing; medical professionals might call it a "mechanical ventilator." Common people may quite often address it as a "breathing machine". It is a bedside mechanism with tubes connected to the airways of patients who need breathing support. It moves breathable air, with some additional oxygen, if required, into and out of the patient's lungs. Fig. (**1**) below shows the mechanical setup of a standard ventilator.

A novel coronavirus has caused the COVID -19 pandemic, a highly contagious disease. The work by Zhu N *et al.* describes it as a highly infectious disease found for the first time at the end of December 2019 in Wuhan, China [3].

Based on the data selected from government health ministries, "The New York Times," and other credible sources, 213 million instances of COVID-19 are reported, with 4.44 million mortalities worldwide.

A study [4] by Iyengar *et al.* (2020) shows how a very mild infection like the common cold or a severe respiratory issue like pneumonia may even lead to the death of the patient.

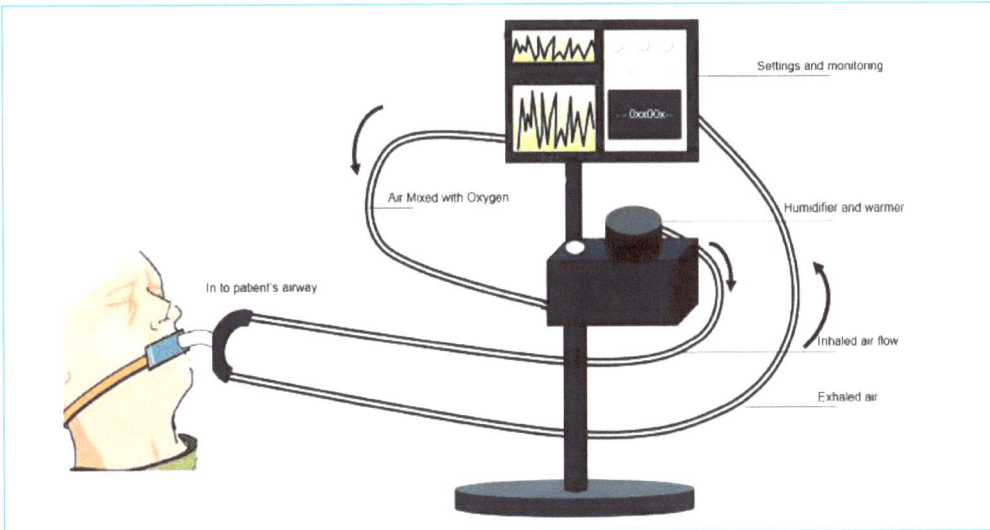

Fig. (1). Illustration of a standard mechanical ventilator setup.

COVID-19 has yet to be treated with a specific treatment., other than having the vaccines produced by different companies across the globe. A ventilator as a lifesaving support equipment is required in many cases to supply air, to the lungs of patients, with an increased amount of oxygen. As a result, one of the most essential pieces of lifesaving equipment is combating the COVID–19 pandemic. COVID-19 patients in critical ICUs requiring ventilator assistance have increased dramatically worldwide. According to a statement released by Imperial College London, 30 percent of COVID-19 patients are projected to require mechanical ventilation support [5].

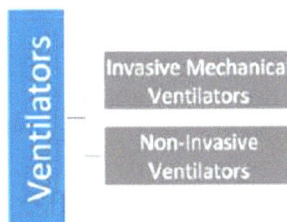

Fig. (2). Categories of ventilators [6].

Ventilators can be basically categorized as Invasive Mechanical Ventilators and Non-Invasive Ventilators given in Fig. (**2**). Invasive ventilators use an endotracheal tube introduced into the trachea to deliver oxygen to the patient's lungs, whilst non-invasive ventilation does not require the use of an internal tube Non-invasive ventilation equipment, including continuous positive airway pressure (CPAP) devices [6] and oxygen hoods, were also used for the management of moderate COVID-19 patients to circumvent the need of intrusive mechanical ventilators. However, mechanical ventilators, are almost often employed when patients have acute respiratory distress syndrome (ARDS), as in COVID-19. This aids in the restoration of normal oxygen levels in the body. They're primarily employed in the care given at home, during emergencies, and critical care set up in hospitals, as well as a component of general anaesthetic equipment.

The resource shortage was apparent. Most of the wealthy nations are being engrossed by a lack of resources which include insufficiency in the number of personal protective equipment (PPE) and ventilators during the pandemic season of (COVID-19) [6]. Governments around the globe have even stated some unethical practices to ensure that the sparse resources are kept for workers in the healthcare system in their own country. Many governments have started negotiating for the complex global supply chain. It is worth noting that nations like Taiwan, Thailand, Russia, and Germany have stopped the export of face masks [7] even during the first half of 2021. Much news said ventilator exports were intercepted during the process and transported to the nations which is making the highest bid. "Modern piracy" could be the best word to describe such a behaviour, written on black pages of history [7]. In addition, there have been allegations of PPE and respiration support devices transportation being intercepted and transferred to the country which can provide more money, which has been dubbed "modern piracy" [7].

Securing breathing devices for patients is undeniably essential in the fight against COVID-19. Many hospitals in developed countries may have an abundant supply of these items; however, most underdeveloped countries were hit severely by the scarcity of such devices.

As scarcity prevails, the death count drastically increases in places where patients in absolute need of critical hospital care are overwhelmed by the availability. Many COVID-19 patients got affected by Acute Respiratory Distress Syndrome (ARDS), a condition that can mainly be treated with mechanical ventilation.

A worldwide shortage of lifesaving ventilators became an international concern, and both big giants in medical equipment engineers and small-scale manufacturers started research into producing emergency respiration machines.

AN OVERVIEW OF 3D PRINTING / ADDITIVE MANUFACTURING

3Dimensional printing is a technique for creating three-dimensional objects' 3D printing, sometimes known as Digital Fabrication Technology or Additive Manufacturing. It is a technique for creating things out of a geometrical model by integrating different materials. It is spreading widely worldwide and is being utilized in sectors such as agriculture, healthcare, aviation, mass customization, and the production of a wide range of equipment and spare parts. 3D printing technology can print an object by depositing material across many layers, one after the other, under direct control by a computer. It has matured to the point that it may use it in various applications. It creates new horizons to give chances to multiple manufacturing organizations looking to improve their efficiency. The materials that can be employed for additive printing are mostly thermoplastics, ceramics, graphene-based materials, and some metals.

3D printing technology /Additive printing can change sectors and bring innovation to the manufacturing process. The utilization of 3D printing technology will undoubtedly increase production speed and thus reduce the cost of production. We should also understand that the customer's demand will have a stronger influence on production. Especially during the final stages of production, the customers will have a greater input to have it produced that fits exactly their requirements and specifications. At the same time, a 3D printer can be located physically closer to the customer, which permits much more flexible and responsive manufacturing. It also gives much flexibility to the quality control process. In addition to that, if we use 3D printing technology, the need for transportation will greatly decrease. This is supported by the fact that when manufacturing sites and the destination location are nearer, transportation required for global distribution can be easily tracked and handled, saving much energy and valuable time.

In any case, 3D printing has its own sets of drawbacks. The most crucial is the loss in the workforce, which has an immediate impact on the economies of countries that rely heavily on low-skilled labour.

Another risky area of the use of 3D printers is the ability of these printers to print potentially dangerous objects like knives, axes, and other things that are potentially harmful to others. Even spare parts for pistols can be easily created using a 3D printer.

As a result, we believe that 3D printing should only be used by individuals who have been granted special authorization so that rebels and terrorists do not have the opportunity to abuse it. If anyone can get hold of the blueprint of a product, they can produce a highly similar counter-feat product without much difficulty. This is especially true now that 3D printing technology is becoming more and more accessible. Give the sketch to the computer, and when the computer issues the command, your 3D printer can swiftly reproduce the sketch.

Additive printing has been widely used in many countries, particularly in manufacturing. In this chapter, I'll go over the several forms of 3D printing, the various materials utilized in manufacturing technologies, and how this can be applied to ventilator manufacture.

For diverse applications, many types of 3D printing have been developed. The ASTM standard F2792 establishes a global standard for additive manufacturing terminology. F2792 was later decommissioned. The new ISO/ASTM 52900:2015 standard was issued in December 2015 and is supported by ASTM and ISO. According to this standard, binder-jetting, Directed Energy Deposition, method of material extrusion, material jetting, powder bed fusion, Sheet lamination and Vat Photopolymerization are key-process categories. The main classification of 3D printing technology is shown in Fig. (**3**). It is not worthwhile to ask which method works best, as each will perform well for the job at hand. We are explaining some of the major 3D printing technologies below.

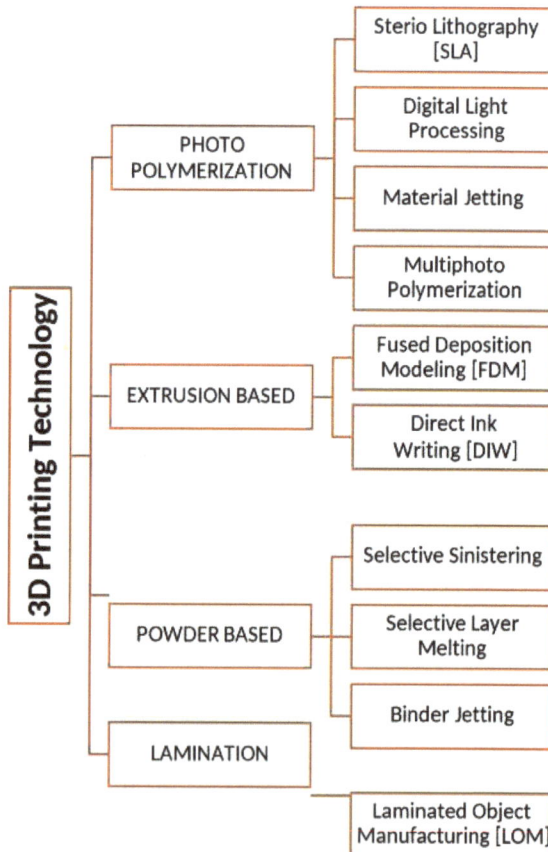

Fig. (3). Some categories of 3D printing technologies [8].

Major 3-Dimensional Printing Technologies

Binder Jetting

This process of 3D printing, called binder jetting, enables rapid prototyping. This method involves selectively depositing a liquid binding agent on top of powder particles to bind them together. Multiple layers of materials are then bonded to obtain the desired object. The binder jetting method forms a layer by spraying a chemical binder onto the dispersed powder. The machine can print metallic, sand, polymer, hybrid, and ceramic materials. Binder jetting is a simple, quick, cost-effective alternative to other printing methods. Binder jetting provides the extra benefit of generating crisp, precise results when printing huge items.

Directed Energy Deposition

The additive printing method is more complicated. This method is typically used to repair or augment existing components. The advantage of this approach is that it may control grain structure to a very high degree. High-quality objects can be created *via* directed energy deposition. Although the Binder Jetting and Directed Energy Deposition processes appear similar, a directed energy deposition printer nozzle is not fixed to a single axis and can travel in any direction. Furthermore, directed energy deposition is beneficial when working with ceramics and polymers. It could also be employed in metals and metal-based hybrids with success. Laser-engineered net shaping is used to illustrate this technology (LENS). This relatively new technology may be used to create or repair things ranging in size from millimetres to meters.

Materials Extrusion

Based on material extrusion, additive printing is particularly suited to printing multi-materials and multi-color polymers, with trials in the realm of printing food and live cells currently underway. This is a widely used approach with meager costs. Furthermore, extrusion materials can be used to make completely functional parts for various products. Fused deposition modelling, or FDM for short, is a good example of this technology. FDM was invented in the early 1990s and a polymer was employed as its primary material. Parts are built one layer after another layer in FDM. The layers are produced by heating and extruding thermoplastic filament from the bottom to the top. Even artificial bones could be printed using this technology. The steps involved in FDM are given below in Fig. (**4**).

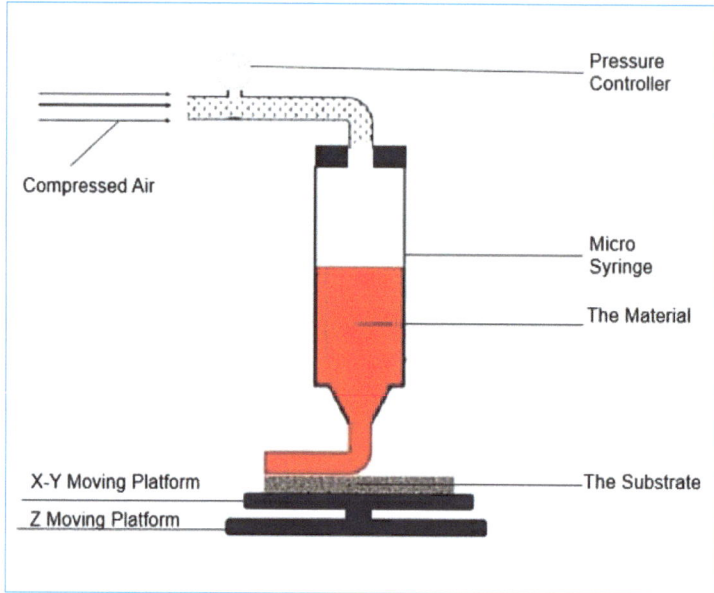

Fig. (4). Material extrusion basic block diagram.

Thermoplastic melted to semi-liquid conditions is then deposited in ultra-fine globules, following the extrusion path.

In case, we need support or buffering during the process, a removable material is deposited, which is strong enough to act as a scaffolding.

Materials Jetting

It is a 3-Dimensional printing procedure. In this technology, construction material is carefully put one drop after drop; as per ASTM Standards here, a print head releases drops of a photosensitive liquid that solidifies and forms a part layer by layer under Ultra-Violet light. Material jetting produces products with a highly polished surface finish and extreme dimensions accuracy simultaneously. Material jetting [8], as shown in Fig. (5) allows multiple material printing to implement an extensive array of stuff like biological agents, polymeric, ceramics, composites, and hybrid materials.

Powder Bed Fusion

Another approach is powder bed fusion, which uses electron beam melting (EBM), SLS, and SHS printing methodologies. We employ either an electron beam or a laser to fuse the material powder. Generally, materials in metals, ceramics, polymers, etcetera are commonly used, though options for composite and hybrid materials are also available. Selective laser sintering (SLS) method is a good illustration of a powder-based additive printing mechanism. In functionality, it is fast-paced, giving good accuracy, and varying texture finishes. Another technology that follows the powder bed fusion is the Selective heat ministering [SHS] technology. A thermal head print is employed for melting the thermoplastic powder to obtain the object *via* additive printing. Fig. (**6**) presents the functionality of Powder-Bed Fusion.

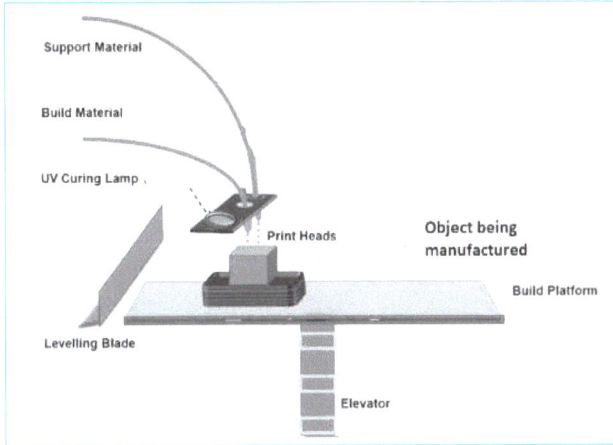

Fig. (5). Material Jetting.

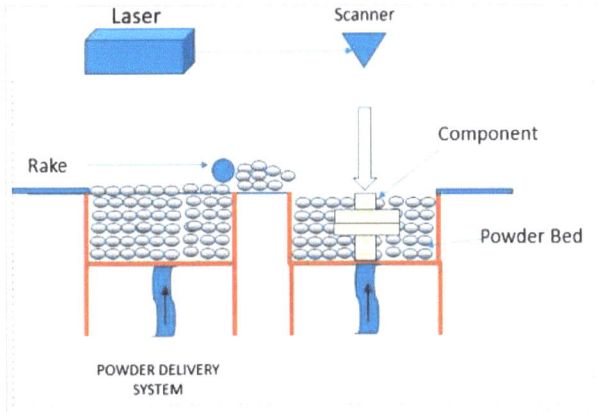

Fig. (6). Powder-Bed Fusion.

Sheet Lamination

As per the specification given by ISO/ASTM, Sheet lamination is an additive manufacturing method wherein material sheets are strongly connected to make a single portion [8]. Laminated Object Manufacturing [LOM] is another name for it. Helisys introduced the LOM technology and in the 1990s, they started manufacturing and selling such machines, which use paper-rolls and laser to make 3D Printed objects.

The LOM is started by laying down a single material layer on the appropriate build surface. The material can be paper, polyvinyl chloride, or metal based on the need and the variety of printers used. This layer will be generally bonded to the previous layers initially and make a 2D cut-through. The multiple layers are bonded together using any of the following methods: glue, melted polymer or atomic migration technique. The 2D cutting can be made using a cutter that uses a very sharp blade, or the cutting can be performed using laser beams. In yet another method, the ceramic tape is cut into required 2D shapes and then stacked one by one on top of each other and put in an oven after applying suitable binders. The material we use determines whether the process is expensive or inexpensive, which then determines which printer is to be used. Fig. (7) presents the general setup needed for Sheet Lamination. Some of the additive printers using this technology use paper rolls as the raw material, which reduces the cost and can even print colour objects efficiently. One disadvantage is that the height of the layer may need to be flexibly changed while keeping the thickness of the used material sheets. LOM can be employed in the additive manufacturing of complicated geometric objects.

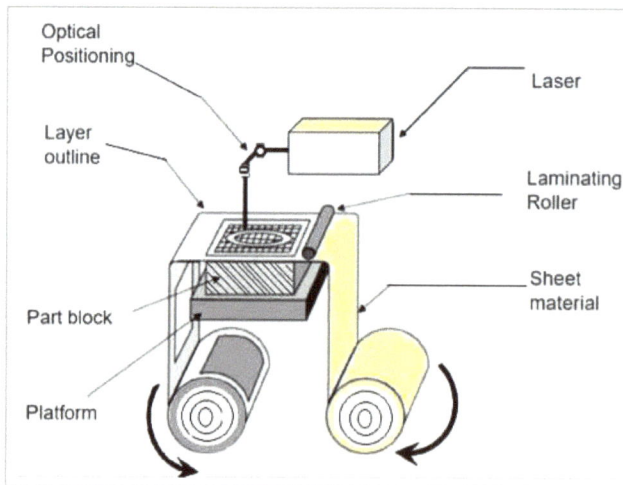

Fig. (7). Basic Illustration of Setup Needed for Sheet Lamination.

Vat Photopolymerization

Vat Photopolymerization is a category of additive manufacturing (3D printing) that can manufacture 3-dimensional objects by selective setting of liquid resin through a targeted light- activated polymerization process. Stereolithography (SLA) and Digital Light Processing are the most popular mechanisms used in Vat

Photopolymerization. A Vat Photopolymerization printer's key attributes are the exposure period, light's wavelength involved and electric supply amount. Initially unique liquid materials are incorporated, which get hardened when exposed to sunlight. The light can vary from ordinary, ultraviolet light or even laser depending on the printer [9].

Common Additive Printing Materials

Similar to all other manufacturing industries, additive printing also needs materials of very high quality to meet consistent quality output objects from the printer. A standard set of procedures, agreements and quality analysis are agreed upon between suppliers and end-users who use the material in their printer. The additive printing can create completely functional parts of a large array of objects including but not limited to Ceramic, metals, polymers and many combinations of them.

Metals

Additive printing technology using metal as the raw material has gained popularity in multiple domains like aeronautical, automobile and medical applications. It should be noted that many metal alloys are usable in building substitution parts for internal organs. Aluminum alloys, cobalt alloys, and titanium are popular in this scenario. This is because metals have specific stiffness, high elastic capacity, and resistance to heat-treated conditions. Titanium alloys are used for printing many biomedical equipment nowadays [9].

Polymers

Polymers are another commonly used material for 3D printing, especially when obtaining objects of highly complex geometry [9, 10]. Fused deposition modelling (FDM) is the most widely used technology when using polymers. Using this concept, we can build additive printer things by layering extruded thermoplastic filaments on each other. Polylactic acid, acrylonitrile butadiene styrene, polypropylene, and polyethene are some of the most popular materials. Thermoplastic filaments with greater melting temperatures have recently been employed as input to additive printers. When choosing a material, liquid polymers or polymers with a low melting point are desirable. Their low weight and low cost make them an attractive target as a raw material for 3D printing.

Ceramics

3D printing has proved its ability to manufacture three-dimensional objects with the help of ceramics and concrete because of the naturally good properties of ceramic materials. Ceramic is considered very strong, and durable and has some good fire-resistant properties. Ceramic objects can be practically built in any geometry and shape, and credit goes to the attributes of ceramics that exist in the fluid state before setting [9, 11]. It is now trendy in building dental applications and aeronautics. Alumina, bioactive glass, and zirconia are good examples of ceramic materials used to create 3D objects.

Composite Materials

Composite materials provide an amazing level of versatility. Most of them are very low weight and tailored based on the need. Industries looking for high performance are keen on composite materials, especially carbon-reinforced polymer composites [9]. The most widely used composite material is polymer composites reinforced with carbon, characterized by stiffness, strength, and resistance to corrosion. Another suitable composite raw material is polymer composite reinforced with glass fibers, characterized by cost-effectiveness and low coefficient thermal expansion.

Other Smart Materials

Those materials capable of altering the geometry and shape based on external conditions like heat or moisture are called intelligent materials [12]. This can be used to design and create self-evolving structures and soft robotic systems. Sometimes they are even referred to as 4D printing stuff. Smart materials used in additive printing include form-memory metals and shape-memory polymers [13]. Shape memory alloys and polymers can be well used in biomedical implants and microelectromechanical devices.

Special Materials

Food, fabric, and other items can be created using additive printing technology when food or fabric components are used as raw materials [9]. Think about children who dislike spinach, funny, lovable shapes can be printed using an additive printer by giving spinach as raw material. Similarly, we can print clothes using nylon or similar things as special raw materials for additive printing.

Application of 3D Printing in the Medical Industry/Healthcare Domain

All these years, the application of 3-Dimensional printing in healthcare has expanded, saving and enhancing lives in previously inconceivable ways. Ophthalmology, cardiology, orthopaedic surgery, heart and lung surgery, neurosurgery, podiatry, oral and maxillofacial surgery, otolaryngology, plastic surgery, pulmonology, oncology, transplantation operations, urology, and vascular surgical procedures have all used 3D printing. Nowadays, a lot of focus is given to additive printing of skin, bone, cartilage, replacement tissues, *etc.* Another important use is the object models printed out for visualization, which helps medical students. The most important aspect is that additive printing can imitate human skin's natural structure at a reasonable cost. Pharmaceutical products, injections, cosmetics, *etc.* can be safely tested on additive-printed skin. Using additive printing technology for printing drugs, the accuracy of dose, and the easy of reproducing the same drug again can be increased. Additive printing can be used to print cartilage and bone, replacing natural bones or cartilage worn or damaged due to accidents or any other illness. It can be employed in restoring and improving tissue functions. This technology benefits cancer-related research as it can form highly controllable cancer tissue mode [14].

Some of the most common applications of 3-Dimensional printing in the medical/clinical domain are listed below.

Preoperative Planning and Tailored Pre-surgical/Treatment

Combining clinical and imaging data will result in a multistep method to find the optimum therapy option. Pre-surgical planning customized to each patient's needs may help reduce operating room time and problems. It also helps reduce post-operative hospitalizations, re-intervention rates, and healthcare costs. The surgeon can obtain a physical 3-Dimensional model of the intended patient anatomy using 3-Dimensional printing technology, which can then be used to propose the surgical plan correctly using cross-sectional imaging or to manufacture customized prostheses (or surgical equipment) based on patient-specific anatomy. This enables a better understanding of complicated anatomy specific to each patient. Furthermore, 3D printing allows surgeons to pick the size of prosthetic components with extreme precision before implantation.

Personalize Surgical Instruments and Prostheses

Additive manufacturing can be utilized to create personalized implants, surgical guides and instruments. As a result of the additive manufacturing process, surgical equipment and prosthesis can be customized at a lower cost.

Research on Osteoporotic Scenarios

After a pharmaceutical treatment, 3D printing can validate the patient's results. This supports a more precise estimation of the subject's bone plus a more informed surgical treatment option.

Enhancing Medical Practice

3D-printed patient-specific prototypes have been shown to improve performance, stimulate rapid learning, and considerably improve student knowledge, management, and confidence, regardless of competence [8]. In comparison to cadaver postmortem, the advantages of 3D printing in pedagogy include the 3-dimensional model's reusability and security. It also supports the ability to represent various physiological and pathophysiological anatomies from a huge image dataset, as well as the capability to distribute 3D models between other organizations, especially those with limited 3D printers capable of printing with the help of various materials. 3D printing with the ability to perform printing of highly dense and different colors can be used to emphasize anatomical intricacies.

Tissue Engineering

Implantable tissue can also be created through 3D printing. One example is the 3D printing of synthetic skin for transplantation to burn sufferers. It can also be used to examine cosmetics, chemicals, and pharmaceuticals. Another example is the replication of human ears utilizing castings full of a gel comprising cartilage cells from cows coated with collagen or the replication of the aortic valve using a merger of cells and polymers to modify the strength of firmness.

Drugs that are Tailored to the Individual

3D printing of medications entails printing out a powdery drug layer for it to dissolve faster than a typical pill.

THE ROLE OF 3D PRINTING, IN MANUFACTURING VENTILATOR COMPONENTS

Until recently, 3D printing, the object creation method in which materials like plastic, ceramic, metal, or composite material layers are stacked to form 3-Dimensional products [15], was mainly used to create prototypes only. However, recent advances made it possible to create original objects using additive printing technology. Especially during this season of the COVID-19 pandemic when the fast creation of many clinical equipment components and spare parts became the need of the hour.

Let's look at some additive printing techniques used to combat COVID-19 in mechanical ventilator parts manufacture.

When fighting a rapidly spreading pandemic like COVID-19, where there is an insufficiency of ventilator machines, one simple but really useful idea proposed was "use of a single ventilator for a cluster of subjects at the same time". The user of splitters could achieve this. A splitter is supposed to divide the airway of one ventilator with the help of a small part named a splitter. In a study [16], the authors suggested the same and successfully created the splitter approved by intensive care specialists. They designed multi-port splitters and manufactured them using 3D printing using a Stratasys J750 printer. They used two sets of splitters, one for inspiration and the other for expiration [16].

Though the designs of ventilator valves, as shown in Fig. (**8**) are subject to patents and copyright, emergencies like the current situation, which cause life-or-death situation, put pressure to make decisions that could justify their full use regardless of thinking about intellectual property acts, especially when done in an appropriate medically approved setting. Isinnova, an Italian startup company, was fruitful in developing steps for manufacturing mechanical ventilator valves to make them available to the local supply. 3-Dimension printed valves saves COVID_19 victims' lives for devices in an Italian hospital [17].

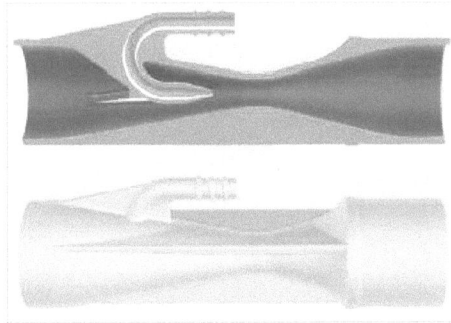

Fig. (8). Design of an Open-source non-adjustable Venturi valve [17].

Another use was to create splitters called T-connectors which would help to use one ventilator for multiple patients. US Food and Drugs Administration (FDA) is not keeping any restrictions on such use of IPR until the emergency declaration period is over.

Multiple ventilators which are fully-automated or semi-automated using flow-driven or pressure controlled safety valves, respiration valves, membranes, *etc.* could be a good target area for 3D Printing. Many manufacturers have reported very promising results.

Albert Chi *et al*. [18] developed and tested a low-cost ventilator using 3D printing technology. It was a flow-driven, pressure-regulated ventilator without any electronic components. They claim that the design can be printed fast and mass-produced at any location based on the need. It should be noted that having a 3D printer and the required materials at the hospital premises is possible. So that the ventilator components can be printed out based on the need, with supervision from the producing company. Reading the salient features of the low-cost CRISIS ventilator developed by Alber Chi and their team is noteworthy. Fig. (**9**) of such a 3D-printed ventilator is given below.

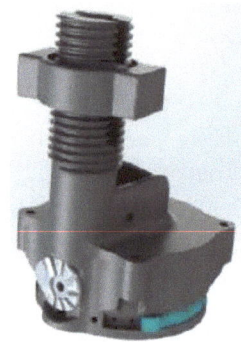

Fig. (9). Crisis Ventilator [18].

The ventilator could be entirely manufactured using off-the-shelf components and a 3D printer.

It reduces the processing time and transportation time due to the supply chain issue.

It does not require any specific speciality manufacturing of spare parts.

It can be created anywhere across the globe.

In India, HP Inc. in partnership with Redington 3D produces ventilator parts. With this initiative, HP has manufactured 12 different components using additive manufacturing techniques and utilized them to manufacture about 10000 ventilators in 2020. The major components which were 3D printed were the valve holders, inhale and exhale connectors, oxygen nozzles, and solenoid mounts; those manufactured ventilators were distributed across different areas of India. It should be noted that they could produce this much number in just 24 days. Across the globe, HP and its partners have printed over 3 million ventilators.

From these, we can understand that 3D printing can be a crucial part of combating COVID-19 or any future pandemic that could cause serious respiratory issues, as it helps manufacture the spare parts or even the entire ventilator. Though the printing may take some time, it is worth enough as there is no need for transportation since the printing can occur in a nearby center or at the hospital where the 3D printer has been installed with sufficient supply or required material. As ceramic, metal, or plastic parts can be printed out using additive manufacturing technology, virtually all ventilator parts can possibly be manufactured. Quality analysis of the printed parts must be done at the manufacturing site. Table **1** below compares 3D printing and conventional manufacturing of ventilator parts in terms of time, quality, flexibility, and material wastage.

Table 1. Comparison of 3D printing with conventional manufacturing for Ventilator parts.

	Additive Manufacturing [3D Printing]	Conventional Manufacturing
Time to create	It may take more time to create a single component, however, this extra time is insignificant as the production of the component can be done at the premises of a hospital thereby reducing the time required for transportation.	During bulk manufacturing, we can produce more objects in a shorter time.
Quality	Need high-quality raw materials, though there is a limitation in the types of items we can use for additive manufacturing, we can select the most appropriate material for each item. Quality checks and quality analysis need to be made from the selection phase of raw materials to the testing of finished products at the site.	Quality Analysis is done by the QA tester after the finished product is available. The product will be sent to market only if it is proven to have the required quality.
Flexibility	Making changes to the shape and geometry of the product is possible and comparatively easy, and the design change is to be made with the software that helps to design the object.	Changing the shape or geometry of an object is comparatively difficult as the change needs to be implemented from the design phase, the moulding phase, till the production checking phase.
Material wastage	As materials are added in consecutive layers, the chances of wastage of material are less.	During the manufacturing, materials are removed from the used row materials, causing an increased chance of wastage of materials

THE ROLE OF 3D PRINTING IN MANUFACTURING COMPONENTS OF OTHER MEDICAL DEVICES

We can manufacture not only the ventilators and ventilator parts with 3D printing technology for combating COVID-19 but also various other objects required for life support or precautionary steps. Some of the examples are explained here.

Face Masks

Quarantine measures in the wake of this disastrous pandemic have caused unbearable tension and fear in the minds of the general public. This caused a phenomenon of panic buying, where people unnecessarily buy things in bulk quantities generating an artificial shortage of these items in the market. This may even cause the unavailability of such materials to the people who need them most, like health care professionals. Though there are multiple challenges, associates of the worldwide 3D printing fraternity have emerged with many ideas for recyclable personal possessions that might be printed using additive manufacturing technologies. As these masks are intended to be reusable, manufacturers must consider the currently available sterilization mechanisms. One advantage of using 3D printers for producing face masks is that we can create custom-size masks after including the option to scan the face of the intended user and implement using computer-aided design [19]. Fig. (**10**) below shows the different mask models

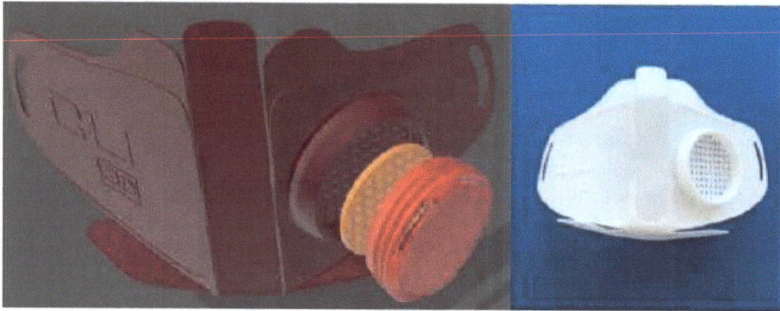

Fig. (10). a) Model of a Copper3D NanoHack mask at an intermediate stage of construction. **b**). The mask as a 3D printed model [20].

Face Shields

"The National Security Innovation Network" (NSIN) [20], which was top spotted by the Dept. of Defense and was effective in printing face shields, gathered up additive manufacturing professionals from all over the world in the USA Unified Production Coalitions. They streamlined the visors' designs to be printed on a 3D printer machine with controlled support of additive materials. Nylon materials or ABS plastics were their favorites. They were able to locate corporate partners with whom they could obtain vast quantities of clear shielding materials.

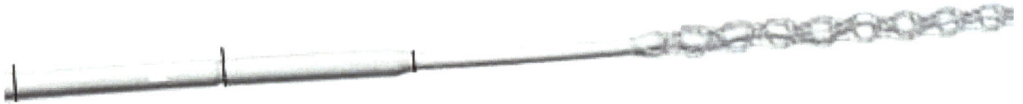

Fig. (11). A 3D printed nasal swab.

Nasal Swabs

The essential approach taken by different countries to combat COVID-19 was to conduct many accurate reverse transcriptase polymerase chain reaction (RT PCR) tests. This is done by collecting respiratory material available in the interior part of our nose. To collect this, we use swabs. A swab is a long stick with a soft cotton-like end. The supply chain of these specimen collection swabs was significantly affected by the pandemic; printing the swabs using 3D printers was a practical solution.

The importance of 3D-printed swabs lies in the number of RT PCR tests done worldwide. The 3D printed swabs (Fig. **11**) designed and produced by the USF Health – North well Health are now abundantly used in the US and worldwide. Many other manufacturers are now manufacturing nasopharyngeal swabs using additive manufacturing technology.

Other Potential Areas

3D-printed orthopaedic implants, scalpels, forceps, other tailored equipment, and individualized dental care objects, are some prospective areas where 3D printing might be implemented in the healthcare domain. Aortic valves, metal hip replacements, coronary stents, and other high-risk medical devices may be printed in the future.

CONCLUSION

Coronavirus illness -19 has wreaked havoc on humanity. We began to think creatively about how to tackle the pandemic. Such imaginative thinking resulted in using 3D printing, also acknowledged as additive manufacturing, to construct products with various intricate dimensions and geometries. As we can see, there was a significant scarcity of ventilation devices and spare parts. Many of the ventilator pieces can now be printed thanks to recent research. The most important benefit was that it allowed for the fabrication of such parts on the grounds of hospitals or healthcare facilities, eliminating transportation and, as a result, decreasing supply chain difficulties and carbon footprint, particularly because transportation was reduced. Aside from mechanical and non-invasive ventilators and their spare components, additive manufacturing is now implemented in the construction of various products using various materials such as polymers, metals, nylon, and composite materials. Face masks of various types, nasopharyngeal swabs for collecting specimens, face shields, syringe pump racks, orthopaedic implants, scalpels, forceps, personalized dental, and other equipment are among the most significant. 3D printing has a lot of applications in healthcare, especially in the event of a future pandemic. We won't have to worry about a severe scarcity of medical or surgical supplies because we can print them locally. There was some leeway for using copyrighted designs during the COVID-19 epidemic. We anticipate that more open-source designs will become available globally, allowing anyone to print lifesaving equipment more quickly at any local hospital. After all, it's a matter of your health.

REFERENCES

[1]   P. Verdecchia, C. Cavallini, A. Spanevello, and F. Angeli, "The pivotal link between ACE2 deficiency and SARS-CoV-2 infection", *European Journal of Internal Medicine,* vol. 76, no. Apr, pp. 14-20, 2020.
[http://dx.doi.org/10.1016/j.ejim.2020.04.037] [PMID: 32336612]

[2]   A.C. Roden, M.C. Bois, T.F. Johnson, M.C. Aubry, M.P. Alexander, C.E. Hagen, P.T. Lin, R.A. Quinton, J.J. Maleszewski, and J.M. Boland, "The spectrum of histopathologic findings in lungs of patients with fatal coronavirus disease 2019 (COVID-19) infection", *Archives of Pathology & Laboratory Medicine,* vol. 145, no. 1, pp. 11-21, 2021.
[http://dx.doi.org/10.5858/arpa.2020-0491-SA] [PMID: 32821902]

[3]   N. Zhu, D. Zhang, W. Wang, X. Li, B. Yang, J. Song, X. Zhao, B. Huang, W. Shi, R. Lu, P. Niu, F. Zhan, X. Ma, D. Wang, W. Xu, G. Wu, G.F. Gao, and W. Tan, "A novel coronavirus from patients with pneumonia in China, 2019", *New England Journal of Medicine,* vol. 382, no. 8, pp. 727-733, 2020.
[http://dx.doi.org/10.1056/NEJMoa2001017] [PMID: 31978945]

[4]   K. Iyengar, S. Bahl, Raju Vaishya, and A. Vaish, "Challenges and solutions in meeting up the urgent requirement of ventilators for COVID-19 patients", *Diabetes & Metabolic Syndrome: Clinical Research & Reviews,* vol. 14, no. 4, pp. 499-501, 2020.
[http://dx.doi.org/10.1016/j.dsx.2020.04.048] [PMID: 32388328]

[5]   S. Eubank, I. Eckstrand, B. Lewis, S. Venkatramanan, M. Marathe, and C.L. Barrett, "Commentary on Ferguson, et al., 'impact of non-pharmaceutical interventions (npis) to reduce COVID-19 mortality and healthcare demand,'", *Bull. Math. Biol.,* vol. 82, no. 4, p. 52, 2020.
[http://dx.doi.org/10.1007/s11538-020-00726-x] [PMID: 32270376]

[6]   M.L. Ranney, V. Griffeth, and A.K. Jha, "Critical supply shortages — the need for ventilators and personal protective equipment during the COVID-19 pandemic", *N. Engl. J. Med.,* vol. 382, no. 18, p. e41, 2020.
[http://dx.doi.org/10.1056/NEJMp2006141] [PMID: 32212516]

[7]   Y.R. Zhou, "The global effort to tackle the coronavirus face mask shortage the conversation", Available at: https://theconversation.com/the-global-effort-(accessed April 10, 2020).

[8]   "Additive manufacturing — General principles — Terminology", Available at: https://www.iso.org/obp/ui/#iso:std:iso-astm:52900:dis:ed-(Accessed on: 20-Jan-2022).

[9]   N. Shahrubudin, T.C. Lee, and R. Ramlan, "An overview on 3D printing technology: Technological, materials, and applications", *Procedia Manuf.,* vol. 35, pp. 1286-1296, 2019.
[http://dx.doi.org/10.1016/j.promfg.2019.06.089]

[10]   S. Saleh Alghamdi, S. John, N. Roy Choudhury, and N.K. Dutta, "Additive Manufacturing of Polymer Materials: Progress, Promise and Challenges", *Polymers (Basel),* vol. 13, no. 5, p. 753, 2021.
[http://dx.doi.org/10.3390/polym13050753] [PMID: 33670934]

[11]   Z. Chen, Z. Li, J. Li, C. Liu, C. Lao, Y. Fu, C. Liu, Y. Li, P. Wang, and Y. He, "3D printing of ceramics: A review", *J. Eur. Ceram. Soc.,* vol. 39, no. 4, pp. 661-687, 2019.
[http://dx.doi.org/10.1016/j.jeurceramsoc.2018.11.013]

[12]   Z.X. Khoo, J.E.M. Teoh, Y. Liu, C.K. Chua, S. Yang, J. An, K.F. Leong, and W.Y. Yeong, "3D printing of smart materials: A review on recent progresses in 4D printing", *Virtual Phys. Prototyp.,* vol. 10, no. 3, pp. 103-122, 2015.
[http://dx.doi.org/10.1080/17452759.2015.1097054]

[13]   A.Y. Lee, J. An, and C.K. Chua, "Two-way 4D printing: A review on the reversibility of 3D-printed shape memory materials", *Engineering (Beijing),* vol. 3, no. 5, pp. 663-674, 2017.
[http://dx.doi.org/10.1016/J.ENG.2017.05.014]

[14]   A. Aimar, A. Palermo, and B. Innocenti, "The role of 3D printing in medical applications: A state of

the art", *J. Healthc. Eng.,* vol. 2019, pp. 1-10, 2019.
[http://dx.doi.org/10.1155/2019/5340616] [PMID: 31019667]

[15]   "3D printing in the battle against COVID-19 emergent materials", Available at:
https://avesis.marmara.edu.tr/yayin/c5ff5d73-a8da-4d99-8495-b58a3bcea99-
/3d-printing-in-the-battle-against-COVID-19(Accessed on: 20-Jan-2022).

[16]   S. Ayyıldız, A.M. Dursun, V. Yıldırım, M.E. İnce, M.A. Gülçelik, and C. Erdöl, "3D-printed splitter
for use of a single ventilator on multiple patients during COVID-19". ", In: *3D Printing and Additive
Manufacturing* vol. 7. , 2020, no. 4, pp. 181-185.

[17]   D. Sher, and M. Perez Colman, "[updating] Italian hospital saves COVID-19 patients' lives by 3D
printing valves for reanimation devices 3d printing media network - the pulse of the am industry",
Available   at: https://www.3dprintingmedia.network/COVID-19-3d-printed-valve-for-reani-
ation-device/.(Accessed on: 20-Jan-2022).

[18]   A. Manero II, P. Smith, J. Sparkman, M. Dombrowski, D. Courbin, P. Barclay, and A. Chi, "Utilizing
additive manufacturing and gamified virtual simulation in the design of neuroprosthetics to improve
pediatric outcomes", *MRS Commun.,* vol. 9, no. 3, pp. 941-947, 2019.
[http://dx.doi.org/10.1557/mrc.2019.99]

[19]   R. Tino, R. Moore, S. Antoline, P. Ravi, N. Wake, C.N. Ionita, J.M. Morris, S.J. Decker, A. Sheikh,
F.J. Rybicki, and L.L. Chepelev, "COVID-19 and the role of 3D printing in Medicine - 3D printing in
Medicine.   Bio.   Med.   Cent",   Available   at:
https://threedmedprint.biomedcentral.com/articles/10.1186/s41205-020-00064-7#Sec1(Accessed on:
20-Jan-2022).

[20]   A. Manero, P. Smith, A. Koontz, M. Dombrowski, J. Sparkman, D. Courbin, and A. Chi, "Leveraging
3d printing capacity in times of crisis: recommendations for COVID-19 distributed manufacturing for
medical equipment rapid response", *International Journal of Environmental Research and Public
Health,* vol. 17, no. 13, p. 4634, 2020.
[http://dx.doi.org/10.3390/ijerph17134634] [PMID: 32605098]

IoT Innovation in COVID-19 Crisis

T. Genish[1,*] and S. Vijayalakshmi[2]

[1] *KPR College of Arts, Science and Research, Coimbatore, India*

[2] *Department of Data Science, CHRIST (Deemed to be University), Pune Lavasa Campus - The Hub of Analytics, Maharashtra 412112, India*

Abstract: The COVID-19 pandemic is a current global threat that surpasses provincial and radical boundaries. Due to the onset of the pandemic disease, the whole world turned entirely in a couple of weeks. Its consequences have come across the personal and professional life of human beings. The current situation focuses on precautions such as wearing a mask, maintaining social distancing, and sanitizing hands regularly. An innovative platform, and smart and effective IoT technology may be applied to follow these steps. This platform fulfills all critical challenges at the time of lockdown situations. IoT technology is more helpful in capturing real-time patient data and other essential information. IoT allows the tracing of infected people and suspicious cases and helps diagnose and treat patients remotely. It also paves the way to deliver essential medical devices and medicines to quarantined places. In the present ongoing crisis, IoT technology is inevitable in monitoring patients infected with COVID-19 through sensors and intertwined networks. The consultations are given to the patients digitally through video conferencing without meeting the medical expert in person. After the diagnosis is made digitally, IoT devices are used to track health data. Smart thermometers are used instead of traditional ones to collect valuable health data and share it with experts. The IoT robots are now a proven technology used for cleaning hospitals, disinfecting medical devices, and delivering medicines, thus giving more time to healthcare workers to treat patients.

Keywords: Agriculture, Artificial intelligence, COVID-19 Pandemic, Cardiovascular, Contact tracing, Computed tomography, Deep Learning, Digital technology, Global positioning system, Healthcare data, IoT technology, IoT robots, Perception layer, Respiration rate, Random forest, Support vector machine, Temperature, Machine learning, Magnetic resonance imaging.

INTRODUCTION

The concept of the "Internet of Things" was revealed by Kevin Ashton to implement RFID-radio frequency identification in supply chain management for

* **Corresponding Author T. Genish:** KPR College of Arts, Science and Research, Coimbatore, India, Tel: +9990353845; E-mail: th.genish@gmail.com

S. Vijayalakshmi, Naveen Chilamkurti, Savita, Rajesh Kumar Dhanaraj and Balamurugan Balusamy (Eds.)

Procter and Gamble [1]. The Internet of Things (IoT) is a powerful technology that connects multiple smart objects in remote network places. Nowadays, IoT technology has transformed hospital-centric healthcare systems into patient-centric healthcare systems [2]. The clinical data can be received from a faraway area with the help of such services hence improving healthcare services' efficiency. In recent years, COVID-19 (Coronavirus Disease 2019), a vast pandemic, has taken away lives, jobs, joy, *etc.* of many people around the world. It is an unprecedented challenge where the entire globe is struggling to come out of this. COVID-19 gets transmitted directly by respiratory droplets through contact with an infected person or indirect contact with contaminated surfaces [3]. Maintaining social distancing, wearing masks and eating a healthy diet are the measures to control the spread of COVID-19. When social space is implemented, it impacts the economy, where it is pronounced more in developing countries. Inequality in income is high in such countries, and economic issues lead to the relaxation of social distancing and thus increase the number of virus-affected cases in Brazil [4]. The patient data about COVID-19 is stored in a cloud and further used for analysis. IoT records the regular activities of COVID-19 patients and warns them of health issues. IoT gives utmost care during this pandemic and improves the livelihood of people. The virus-affected patients with health complications such as asthma, diabetes, blood pressure, lung infection, *etc.* are monitored effectively by intelligent medical equipment. The equipment is linked to a smartphone to effectively communicate essential medical information to the doctors. It also captures important information on weight, sugar level, oxygen level, *etc.* Accurate and trustworthy medical information are the major problems in healthcare during COVID-19, and IoT settled this issue. IoT offers industries a market to fight effectively with COVID-19 and accelerate the healthcare systems' digitalization. Further developments in IoT could predict future pandemics by applying statistical methods and incorporating artificial intelligence (AI) and big data.

IOT TECHNOLOGY IN COVID-19

Since late 2019, the globe has been fighting a new Coronavirus disease spread in China by severe respiratory syndrome [5]. In March 2020, WHO (World Health Organization) announced the disease as a pandemic since more cases have been registered worldwide. There were about 21,991,954 cases by August 2020 [6]. The disease was spreading significantly faster among human beings. Common symptoms of this disease are fever, sore throat, dry, and respiratory problems. Most people have faced symptoms at a very low level, but people who have an illness or are over 60 years of age have a high risk of death. Government organizations have made several efforts to stop the further spread of COVID-19 and find a vaccine. Most efforts are made to develop a medicine for coronavirus and find ways to control its spread. Hence, there is a considerable demand for monitoring virus-affected patients globally. Currently, IoT has been playing a significant role in healthcare systems, where it helps in different phases of diseases. IoT becomes feasible to achieve effective prevention and control of COVID-19 with the support of other emerging technologies such as AI, big data, and fog computing. An IoT-established system [7] is implemented during COVID-19. In this platform, a computing architecture is adopted consisting of four layers: perception layer, networking layer, fog layer, and cloud layer.

Perception Layer

The perception layer is implemented in homes, hospitals, or outdoors to collect all types of data, such as symptoms or vital signs of human activities, with the help of IoT sensors. Various sensors in the perception layer receive data in the surrounding environment and individuals. These IoT sensors investigate human activities and non-clinical healthcare. The layer consists of the following devices.

Camera–It is an essential and commonly used sensor in IoT devices. The camera captures image and video data. Data collected from the camera are analyzed for COVID-19, *i.e.,* non-contact monitoring and identifying human activities.

Internal sensor – It is a sensor that is built into smartphones and wearable devices such as accelerometers and gyroscopes. An accelerometer measures the acceleration along three axes. From the acceleration measurements, a device's dynamic force, such as vibrations, gravity and movement, are detected. Gyroscope, another sensor, has a rotating wheel with three axes of rotation. It measures the position and talks about how the device is tilted. Attributes of human behaviors are obtained from the readings of this internal sensor.

Magnetometer– Another important IoT sensor that detects magnetic fields along the perpendicular axes. Information from the magnetometer is applied to screen contact tracing and social distancing.

Microphone– It is an acoustic sensor that measures ambient sound signals. Recent IoT devices are made up of MEMS - micro-electro-mechanical systems. MEMS provides SNR - high signal-to-noise ratio and consumes low power. Most research utilizes microphones for the recognition of human activities. A microphone is used along with speakers to transmit acoustic and reflected signals.

Commodity WiFi–To facilitate sensing, the measurements of WiFi such as RSSI - Received Signal Strength Indicator and CSI - Channel State Information are used. During the propagation of WiFi signals, the attenuation is characterized by RSSI.

RSSI is an unstable one that can be easily affected by environmental changes. CSI describes how a signal is propagated from a transmitter to a receiver.

mmWave RADAR – It explores to make non-contacting and non-invasive monitoring. It modulates signals to a particular frequency range and derives the movements of objects using reflected signals. Unlike RSSI, the radar is very robust to changes in the environment. For instance, sound and light do not disturb the sensing power of mm-wave radar. It is preferably installed in most IoT devices as it can achieve a high range of accuracy in the recognition of human activities.

Radio Frequency Identification (RFID) – is a technology that can recognize an exact target by radio signals. The components of RFID are the reader, tag, and antenna. The reader is connected with another reader to broadcast data within a tag. Then the radio signals will be identified from the tag by the reader. The chip, a coupling element, and small antenna are the tag's components and the antenna's role is to get a signal from the reader. A unique code is attached to an object inside the tag to identify the target object.

Network Layer

It is the connecting layer that connects the perception and middleware layers. The network layer collects data from the perception layer and passes it to the middleware layer using technologies such as 4G/5G, satellite networks, WiFi, UTMS, infrared, *etc*. The network layer is also referred to as a communication layer, as it is responsible for connecting the perception and middleware layer. The data in the network layer is transferred more securely and confidentially.

The datagram from the transport layer is encapsulated into data packets at this layer using IP addressing. IPv4 is a standard protocol for the network layers, but has limited address space to cope with the applications of IoT. IPv6 protocol is now developed to accomplish sufficient address space for millions of IoT devices. The popular network layer protocols used in IoT are IPv4, IPv6, 6LoWPAN, 6TiSCH, *etc*.

Fog Layer

The Fog infrastructure is a methodology developed in Cisco [8] where the data, computation, storage, and applications are placed between the cloud and the data source. Data gathered from IoT devices are transferred from the fog layer to the corresponding node for the application's –real-time data analysis. The node enables functions such as compute, store and connectivity. Fog computing has decentralized devices which can perform various functionalities to support mobility. Location-sensitive and time-sensitive NPIs (non-pharmaceutical interventions) are implemented in the fog layer [9] for COVID-19 symptom identifications, quarantine screening, social distancing, and contact tracing.

Cloud Layer

The layer receives information through the microcontroller and then stores data in API (Application peripheral interface). Cloudflare supports infrastructure and applications and safeguards all the info with a built-in firewall. In addition, data about patient symptoms, location, and emergency contact reside in Cloudflare's global network. API exchanges SMS/Email alerts to the family members, relatives, or friends of COVID-19 patients in case of an emergency. The centralized server data centre resides in this layer which has the capabilities of information processing and high storage capabilities. The fog layer is unable to handle the task of predicting complex events. Here, the fog layer is replaced with the cloud layer, which has robust computing capabilities. The cloud layer is implemented with robust big data and deep learning strategies for the system's performance.

APPLICATIONS OF IOT-ENABLED DEVICES

In a complex situation, the patients need to be connected and screened by medical experts in several phases, such as early symptoms diagnosis, time of quarantine, and after recovery. In phase 1, faster virus diagnosis is more important, where the affected person can easily transform the virus into other people. When the diseased patient gets a fast diagnosis, the rate of spread can be in control at the right time, and the patient can get additional treatment. IoT devices are used in this scenario to fasten the process of virus detection by measuring body temperature. Quarantine time is an essential period during COVID-19 in which the affected person should be isolated for treatment. During this phase, IoT devices monitor patients remotely [10]. CDC - Centers for Disease Control and Prevention reported that people with very mild symptoms may recover by staying at home. They don't need any treatments, but they may be infected again after recovery. The people may get the infection again with different symptoms. One of the treatments during this phase is maintaining social distance. Social distancing is followed by deploying IoT devices such as bands and crowd-screening devices. They are applied to track people and ensure social distancing. The devices such as drones, wearables, IoT buttons, and robots are used to fight COVID-19.

A new IoT system is employed to monitor patients' health using the components like sensors, microcontrollers, cloud-enabled systems, and actuators [11]. It can measure the health status of the COVID-19-infected person and physiological parameters and sends the health information to (API) that screens for the level of infection. It comprises 3 layers: wearable layer, cloud layer, and web frontend layer. Each layer is interconnected with others to share and monitor COVID-19 patients remotely.

Wearables

The wearable is a technology that combines electronics and other devices that can be worn. Wearable is a computing technology that can receive and process input when worn to the body as a band, glass, and watches. It is designed to apply in different domains such as healthcare, lifestyle, *etc.* These devices cover several wearable components namely smart helmets, smart thermometers, smart glasses, EasyBand and IoT-Q-Band. Wearable sensor alerts physiological changes like heart rate, variations in heart rate, and respiration rate. These metrics are the important markers of COVID-19. Wearable devices also report complex metrics like stress, activity, recovery, and sleep. Such metrics are measured from the combination of cardiac and accelerometer metrics. IoT-based tools for preventing and controlling COVID-19 are listed in Table **1**.

Table 1. IoT tools used to prevent and control Coronavirus.

Challenges During COVID-19	Applications of IoT in Screening Patients	Perception Layer
Diagnosing COVID-19 symptoms	Breathing	Inertial sensor
		Microphone
		Mm Wave radar
		Depth camera
		WiFi
	Body temperature	RFID
		Infrared temperature sensor
		IRT camera
	Blood oxygen saturation	PPG sensor
		Oximeter
		RGB camera
Quarantine Monitoring	Tracking human activities and contacts	RFID
Contact tracing & Social distancing		Motion sensor
		Drone
		GPS
		WiFi, Bluetooth

(Table 1) cont.....

Challenges During COVID-19	Applications of IoT in Screening Patients	Perception Layer
Outbreak forecasting	Disease prediction	Smartphone and body sensor
		Wearable device
		GPS

Cardiovascular Monitoring

HR (Heart rate), HRV (Heart rate variability), and heart rhythm are the metrics for cardiac functions. The changes in such metrics are the indications of coronavirus infection. Viral infections in the body make HR higher. In the case of a viral infection, increased HR can be identified within an hour or days before the symptoms. Researchers have recently released a study called DETECT -Digital Engagement and Tracking for Early Control and Treatment. This research reveals the changes in HR as a result of COVID-19. Application called myData Helps is used to assess HR, sleep, and activity data from 100000 individuals. The application uses Fitbit, Apple Watch, and Garmin Watches coupled with Google Fit, Apple Health and Amazefit platforms. Stanford University researched that changes in skin temperature can be utilized for predicting COVID-19 before the symptoms. ECG and PPG are mainly applied in wearable sectors for monitoring cardiac functions. ECG shows electrical activities in the heart, and PPG is to measure changes in the blood volume level by using light waves. ECG sensors are implemented to study stratum corneum, and wrist-worn sensors monitor heart rhythms from wearables like Apple Watch. PPG is being measured continuously in several body parts, including fingertips, wrist, earlobes, *etc.*

Cardiovascular Sleep and Activity

Most wearable devices show users data on stress, sleep, and activity. The combination of these measurements is taken daily for the prediction of COVID-19. Cardiovascular stress is derived from the combinations of HR and HRV measurements. Cardiovascular strain will be high when the patient is affected by a viral infection. Viral infections like COVID-19 increase stress on the cardiovascular system reflected by indicators such as HR, RHR, and stress hormone known as catecholamines. Sleep is calculated by combining HR and accelerometer data. The measurements of HR and HR assess the quality of sleep, but an accelerometer may be used to calculate disturbances in sleep. Activity on a day is measured based on physical efforts on the day. Elevated HR and accelerometry measure activity score.

Respiration Monitoring

Respiration rate (RR) plays a key role in COVID-19, where the virus causes severe effects on the lungs. The lower respiratory tract infection by coronavirus declines the overall functions of the lungs and leads to respiration problems. The current guidelines recommend that the measurement of RR can be used as a parameter for intensive care unit (ICU) admissions. RR is received from wearable sensors which compute heart activities due to Respiratory Sinus Arrhythmia (RSA). CovIdentify is an application designed by Duke University that uses devices like Fitbit to monitor an individual's activities, such as oxygen level, sleep schedule, and activity level, to determine the risk of COVID-19. When such data is obtained, predictive algorithms are applied to find respiratory problems from the coronavirus.

Temperature Monitoring

Temperature is a common metric used by several countries to detect COVID-19. Quarantining the infected patients may prevent the transmission of infection to some extent because COVID-19 can be developed before fever starts. Skin temperature on the body is monitored continuously with the help of wearable devices such as VivaLNK Scout and TempTraq. The change in body temperature is combined with HRV and RHR data and can be further used to predict coronavirus before symptoms arise. The skin temperature monitoring wearable can also track fever and alert patients and medical persons.

ROLE OF DRONES TO COMBAT COVID-19

During the COVID-19 pandemic, drone technology was built in several countries. It has been identified that there are three important use cases of drones in response to COVID-19. They include i. pick-up of the samples from the lab, delivery, and transportation of medicines – to minimize the transportation time and the exposure to getting infected, ii. Aerial spraying – to spray in contaminated areas and iii. Monitoring social distance and guidance during quarantine. A drone is simply an aircraft that can fly without human operations. It is also referred to as an "unmanned aerial vehicle" - UAV. The drone concept came in the 1849 war between Italy and Austria, filled with bombs. It uses sensors, Global Positioning System (GPS), and communication services. The IoT, implemented as the Internet of Drone Things (IoDT) allows drones to perform tasks like searching, monitoring and delivering [12]. The drone consumes less energy, takes minimum time, and can run by smartphones and controllers. Drones are applied efficiently in healthcare, agriculture, and the military. Several kinds of IoT-based drones, including medical, disinfectant, thermal imaging, and surveillance, have been used in the combat of COVID-19.

Aerial Spraying and Monitoring of Crowds

Spraying a disinfectant in public places or crowded areas is an effort to control the spread of coronavirus. Normally, the spraying is performed manually, but it leads to uneven spraying, consumes more time, and requires a huge number of human resources. An automatic spraying technology called a drone is the only remedy to resolve this problem. The architecture of drones integrates internal processes to become more efficient due to the design and development of AI. Cloud computing technologies are then used for storing data. The data handling is employed from a nearby location to distant places. Drones are being utilized in all ways to fight COVID-19. They are designed to spray pesticides in crowded public places (shown in Fig. **1**) and in contaminated zones as the cases of COVID-19 rise. A few scenarios where drones are effectively used during COVID-19 are explained as follows:

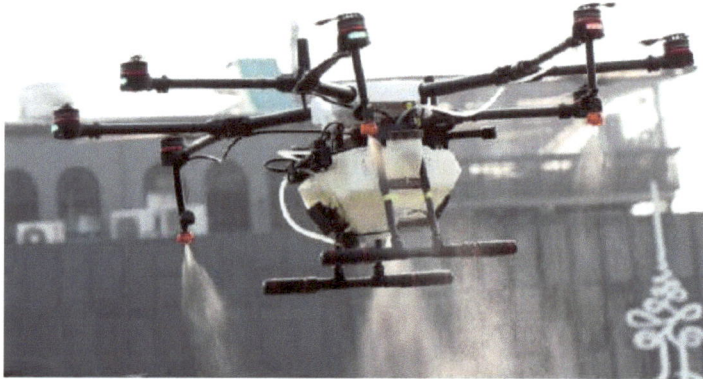

Fig. (1). Drone is spraying disinfectants in public areas.

In Australia, a drone is designed to detect a person who faces problems in their respiratory system. The drone sensor records a person's body temperature, heart pulse rate, and respiratory function by calculating the respiration rate and other abnormalities in the human body. Such measurements are taken from public places where there is more crowd. The technology is being applied now for monitoring people and medication. The technology becomes effective as it saves the lives of human beings working in critical infrastructure. The MicroMultiCopter Company of China has used 100 drones for surveillance over many cities. The drones are alarming people if the inter-personal distance has been failed to maintain. It also gives an alarm when people are walking without wearing a mask. The same scenario is followed in Spain and UAE. In India, government officials have given provisions to the police department to apply drone technology for medication, monitoring, sanitizing, data analysis, and decision-making. Higher officials are monitoring the situations from the control stations and taking some preventive measures.

According to the reports by the Indian Institute of Science, Bengaluru, it is found that the area covered by drones to spray disinfectants is six times more compared to manual spraying. Neel Sagar, the founder of Alpha Drone Technology, has deployed six hexacopter drones that can operate 6-7 hours daily. A single battery can power a drone for about 25 minutes. It covers an area of 6 m/s.

Indian Institute of Technology (IIT) - Guwahati has designed a drone that automatically sanitizes large places, roads, and malls to control the spread of COVID-19. The drones have accomplished their task in less than 15 minutes, which will take 1.5 days of work if done manually. Students claimed that the drones would also be used to record videos and that one operator controls the sprayer option and its activities can be monitored by another operator. The roads and places to be sanitized are selected on Google Maps, and the drone performs the task within a range of 3 kilometers. It covers about 1.2 hectares in one trip and 60 hectares in a single day.

Cargo Delivery

Researchers in Sweden have modelled a cargo drone to tackle a novel coronavirus. It allows drones to distribute tests to the people and collect the test reports back to the laboratories. The test result is then informed to the people electronically so that those who receive positive results can put themselves into quarantine. The team then models optimum drone routes based on the capacity of drones that can fly 12 hours per day at a speed of 37 miles per hour.

Drone Delivery Canada (DDC) transported cargo drones to Beausoleil First Nation (BFN) community in Ontario. It can carry about 10 pounds of the payload and will fly in a defined two-way delivery route of about 3 miles. Totally, 36 drones are built, each carrying 100 tests and may visit every one in a city population of 100000 inhabitants repeatedly every four days. The delivery includes test swabs, hygiene kits, and personal protective equipment (PPE). The cargo drone with the test swabs and other kits is shown in Fig. (**2**). In the study, the researchers integrated a model of a drone-based test kit with a standard susceptible-infected recovered model.

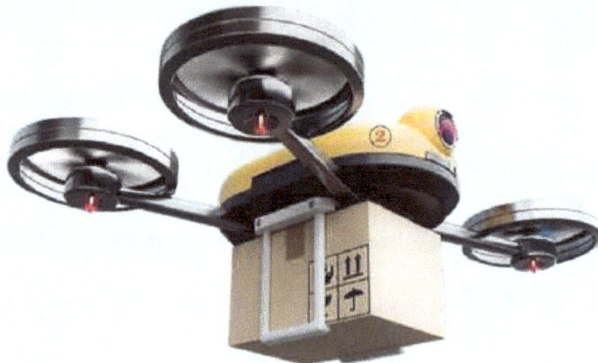

Fig. (2). Cargo delivery drone.

Temperature Scanning

Drones have been utilized during the pandemic to detect fever. During 2002-2004, thermal image technology was used by several Asian countries during the SARS outbreak. The drones now have the same features and created aerial monitors to collect health data through computer vision. Drone technology is being employed in countries such as India, Oman, the US, Italy, and China. A Chinese company Alibaba, offers a drone through Artificial Intelligence (AI) systems that can detect COVID-19 infection with an accuracy rate of 96%. Draganfly, a Canada-based company, claims its pandemic drone can measure temperature, heart, and respiratory rates using sensors and computer vision systems. Draganfly reports that the drone has also been equipped to detect sneezing and coughing of people in crowded places.

According to the report of UNICEF, countries such as Ghana, Rwanda, Sierra Leone, Malawi, and several others have foundations to mobilize the technology instantly from the onset of the pandemic. Even though there is a lack of evidence of the drone's impact on health, these countries can design drones due to factors such as skills, regulation, capacity, resources, *etc.* The framework given by the UNICEF Supply Division provides systematic guidance for the countries to determine the utilization of drones during a pandemic. The framework is based on a decision tree that outlines important steps and components of drone delivery integration. By observing the current situation, the UNICEF Supply Division listed some of the reasons hindering the scalable, widespread and efficient drone deployment.

Lack of Understanding of the Use Case, Problem, and Scenario where Drones can add More Value During the COVID-19 Pandemic

It is shown in the experience that every use case is problem-specific. Therefore, drones' impact and potential benefits in logistics especially, in development and humanitarian contexts cannot be generalized. For instance, transportation time is declined by 70%, as shown in the report by the implementers of drone delivery projects in China. But it does not show sufficient evidence for impact. Similarly, Ghana offers some advantages in its drone technology. It shows that the drone operation reduces the turnaround time but it remains unclear how it contributes to the entire supply chain in rural health facilities where drones fail to offer bi-directional transportation.

Lack of Support Systems

The drones have been used in a limited number of cases during a pandemic, suggesting that they are limited to pilot projects and short time initiatives. When time plays a key role, the responders and agencies may focus on traditional methods to handle the situation rather than experimenting with new technologies. Besides identifying use cases, the drone mechanism depends on whether the trained personnel are available to activate the drones immediately. It depends on procurement and operational deployment plans, which enable drones quickly in emergencies for applications such as aerial spraying, transport, and mapping.

ROBOTIC TECHNOLOGY DURING PANDEMICS

Robotic technology minimizes human contact to control the transmission rate of coronavirus. It is designed to deliver medical things, sanitation, patrolling, and monitoring. Robotics is an interdisciplinary research of computer science and engineering. The ultimate aim of robotics is to design machines that can work and act like humans. Robotic technology was developed to fulfill the requirements of human resources in several developed countries. They are used in various applications such as healthcare, agriculture, manufacturing, underwater exploration, food preparation, *etc.* In healthcare, robotic surgery allows physicians to conduct the clinical and surgical procedures from any part of the world without touching the patient. Arthrobot was the first surgical robot that followed voice commands to help position during a surgical case. AESOP - Automated Endoscopic System for Optimal Positioning was the first robot used for surgery and got approval from FDA - the Food and Drug Administration of the United States in 1996. It used ZEUS, a robotic system with seven degrees of freedom, motion scaling, and tremor elimination. ZEUS was used for long-distance surgical procedures. Here, laparoscopic cholecystectomy was done on a French patient while the surgeon was available in New York. Surgical care is an important foundation of the healthcare system that contributes more to the needy. During this pandemic, operating rooms can be a high risk for medical society for COVID-19 transmission.

The current COVID-19 pandemic creates several threats to the entire humanity. Several types of robots have been utilized potentially in healthcare to face the challenges of this huge pandemic. In addition to the threats, governments and medical staff in all the countries have faced shortages of personal protective equipment (PPE). Another important factor is limited workforce. The robots can help societies from both factors, i. by reducing the contact between medical staff and patients and ii. serving at the maximum during this pandemic.

The COVID-19 emergency in early 2020 caused many companies to design a robot. Robot-making companies receive huge orders from governments, hospitals, and other organizations. A robot does not need to wear masks, can be disinfected, and will never get sick. Robots can monitor patients, sanitize hospitals and give assistance to hospital workers. UBTech Robotics of China uses robots with a thermal camera in its head to measure body temperature and remind people to wash their hands and wear masks. To fasten COVID-19 testing, Danish doctors at the University of Southern Denmark designed a fully automatic swab robot. They are built using machine learning and deep learning to locate the target area in the throat. The robotic arm gathers samples from the throat with complete consistency, which humans can't attain. Esben Ostergaard, CEO at REInvest Robotics, Denmark, and one of the creators of this fully automatic robot, put his neck on the robot to demonstrate that it is safe.

UVD (UV Disinfection) Robots developed a robot that uses laser light. It was developed after six doctors from Sassarese Hospital, Italy infected with COVID-19. One of the important applications of robotics in this pandemic is to disinfect hospital rooms and surrounding areas with ultraviolet radiation. The users should be aware of the limitations of UV light. The machine carries powerful short-wavelength UV-C (ultraviolet-C) light which destroys the virus's genetic material after exposure. UV-C kills pathogens on the surface of the air. At the same time, it is hazardous to the human beings. Radiation exposure to UV-C is why it is used in autonomous or semi-autonomous mobile robots. A robot called 'humanoid' was developed by Diligent Robotics for a hospital in Texas. The humanoid can bring medicines to the patient's rooms, as shown in Fig. (3). It does this task day and night continuously to allow medical staff to interact more with the patients.

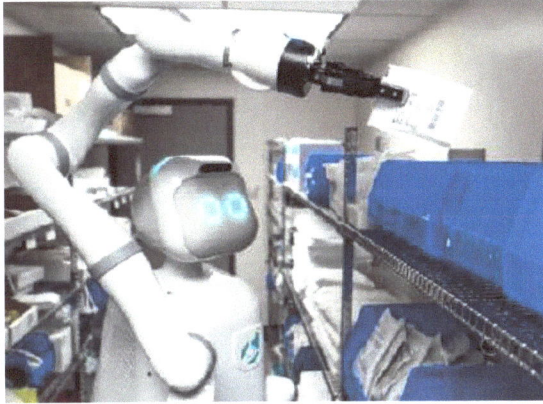

Fig. (3). Humanoid robot fetches medicines from Lab.

Northern Italy suffered a lot due to COVID 19, where the government, non-government organizations, doctors, and nurses faced various challenges. Circolo Hospital, Varese, uses robots to monitor its patients around the clock. Robots designed by Sanbot are armed with cameras and microphones to collect patients' health data, such as blood oxygen levels.

Mitra (meaning 'friend' in Hindi), a robot used at Fortis Hospital, Bangalore, India, to screen COVID-19 patients. Mitra has been employed with facial recognition technology with a tablet in its chest, which allows patients and their family members to look at each other (Fig. **4**). It is a product developed by Bangalore startup Invento Robotics. It is very popular among Indian hospitals as its cost is lower than $13,600, and it is efficient in handling the pandemic. It lowers the risk of COVID-19 to the doctors and medical staff. Mitra was initially designed to care for homes. Then was being adapted to hospital applications during the time of the pandemic. In a clinical application, it helps medical people while taking vital readings. Also, it gives a consultation making Mitra exported to various countries such as Australia, the United States and others. Data analysis and processing are the key factors in the healthcare domain being automated after the pandemic. In a traditional method, the hospital staff manually records the patient's data into the computer. After the entry of robots in healthcare, the healthcare networks connect their patient-facing medical equipment to the cloud allowing the patient's data to be tracked automatically.

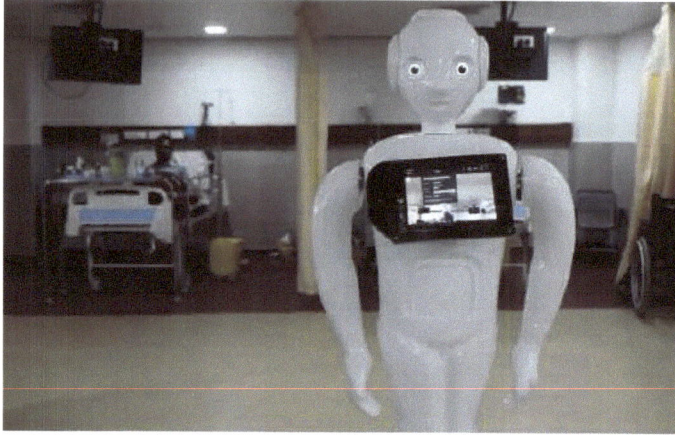

Fig. (4). Mitra is being used for the interactions of patients and their loved ones.

Growth of the Robotics Market

According to the reports given by Business Standard in 2018, India will become a leading robotics manufacturer, and its market is expected to increase by about 20% between the years 2017 and 2025. The International Federation of Robotics (IFR) says that four million industrial robots could be used in 2022 globally to speed up the economy, which has decreased the COVID-19 outbreak. It does not mean that robot replaces workers, but it confronts everyone. It improves the operations and production of an industry with consistent quality. Post-COVID paves a way to contribute new inventions in the deployment of robots. Industries have started implementing robotics technology for their sustainability and growth, as getting skilled laborer is challenging. Robot in the industry ensures three factors such as i. reduces the risk of disruptions during production ii. monitors social distancing in the workplace, and iii. reduces contact between humans and products.

Robotics After COVID-19 Pandem*ic*

Automated robots and devices have changed the scenario of industry in recent years. Garment industry and food industries also started using robots to do work. Warehouse and manufacturing robots were become more popular. Big corporate companies like Amazon, Flipkart, *etc.* started delivering through robots and drones. Meanwhile Tesla introduces the next level of autopilot in e-cars. Innovations made human work easier but people lost their jobs. In the future, more jobs must be needed for this exponentially increasing population.

APPLICATIONS OF AI AND DIGITAL TECHNOLOGY IN COVID 19

AI is a potential technology that helps us to fight with coronavirus. It improves the understanding of the disease, planning, treatment, and test results. The application of AI allows physicians to focus on the treatment and the control of coronavirus. It can diagnose the disease from the images taken by CT - Computed tomography and MRI - Magnetic resonance imaging (MRI). The most important applications of AI during COVID-19 are listed below.

Healthcare

Healthcare industries use AI in addition to robotics to control the transmission of coronavirus. AI helps analyze Computed Tomography (CT) scans, allowing doctors to decide about COVID-19. CT helps diagnose coronavirus infection faster than the standard method RT-PCR (Reverse Transcription Polymerase Chain Reaction). Even though CT provides results faster than RT-PCR, radiologists need more time to analyze CT images. It leads to more workload for a doctor when many COVID-19 cases are considered. AI ensures a patient's health and even detects people with certain symptoms of COVID-19. It improves the efficiency of medical staff and reduces the diagnosis time. Reports of Beijing Infervision Technology, Ping A Smart Healthcare, and the Ministry of Digital Economy and Society, Government of Thailand, revealed that the systems built with AI technology can analyze CT images more efficiently. AI interprets a CT image consistently with an accuracy rate of 90%, thus reducing the time consumed for diagnosis and workload.

In Royal Bolton Hospital, run by the National Health Service (NHS) of the UK, patients often need to wait more than six hours for a radiologist to look at the patient's x-rays. To address this problem, qXR, an AI-based chest x-ray system, has been designed by the Mumbai-based company Qure.ai. The plan was checked for more than six months and finally approved. This system can find the lung abnormalities of COVID-19 patients. During the initial stage of coronavirus, there occurred delays in PCR tests, and hence this chest X-ray system became one of the fastest and most affordable ones for radiologists.

Diagnosis of coronavirus is trickier as the symptoms also resemble those of other diseases. Scientists in New York designed an AI system that can diagnose patients with COVID-19 using an AI algorithm. The algorithm has been trained with more than 900 CT scans of the lungs. Trained with lung scans alone is insufficient because the scan appears normal in the early stage of COVID-19 and lung problems. To address this problem, the AI system was rebuilt, which cross-references CT scans of a patient with additional data such as age, symptoms, and possible contact with the virus. The system produced promising results as it diagnosed seventeen out of twenty-five patients with COVID-19 positive though their CT scans looked normal. Another AI framework was developed by MIT researchers that can detect COVID-19 from the sound they produce when coughing. The team developed an algorithm that gets audio input from thousands of coughs and self-reported the information.

Detecting COVID-19 Cases in Public Areas

AI technology has been applied during this pandemic not only for the medical care workers' welfare but also to identify potential COVID-19 patients in public places. It is achieved by integrating an AI system with infrared technology that allows screening of an individual's body temperature since the common symptom of COVID-19 is fever. SenseTime, a leading AI giant, has deployed a 'Smart AI Epidemic Prevention Platform' with the help of computer vision and deep learning. This platform is implemented in various places in China to regulate the spread of the virus. The Artificial intelligence system promises fast and effective monitoring and detection of suspected people in public places. The system has been extended to schools, community centers, and subway stations in the cities like Beijing and Shanghai. The robust design can scan up to 10 people per second and detect individuals remotely with fever symptoms. Smart AI Epidemic Prevention Platform can detect a fever with an accuracy of $\pm\ 0.3°$ C and identifies people who are not wearing a face mask with a success rate of 99%. At Beijing Airport station, the system allows passengers to move through the security checkpoint directly without a manual temperature check.

In addition, SenseTime has deployed another AI system known as SenseMeteor Smart Commute, which is being installed in the public subway systems in China. It allows new payment methods using face recognition and QR codes. The system is implemented on existing tickets, thus minimizing potential virus transmission. The system provides passengers with an alternative contactless physical payment. It allows them to login into the metro apps, complete the preregistration process and use their faces or QR code to enter the subway. The fare is automatically deducted through pre-set pay mode. The hands-free ticketing system avoids the physical handling of cash and helps reduce the risk of virus transmission.

Contact Tracing

Conventionally, human involvement is needed for contact tracing. If any patients test COVID-19 positive, government officials and health investigators monitor the movement of the patient's contact within a certain time and notify all the contacts manually. It is a tedious job when the infected persons are high because their contact history is also high. To address this inconvenience, technology comes with digital implementations that can monitor the movement of patients through their mobile phones. Singapore released an app called TraceTogether that adopts Bluetooth technology to help health officials screen contact tracing. Aarogya Setu is an app developed by the Ministry of Electronics and IT, India, to help people identify the risk of contracting coronavirus. After installing the app, the user must always switch on Bluetooth and location. The user is asked multiple questions like name, age, contact number, and countries visited in the last thirty days. The information is stored in a government server, and a unique digital id (DiD) will be hashed. When the two registered users are supposed to come within their Bluetooth range, the app exchanges their digital and notes the time and location of the contact. If a registered user results COVID-19 positive, the data is securely uploaded from the user's mobile and stored on the server. Then this data is used for contact tracing and identifies all the persons who have close contact with the infected person.

China introduced health QR codes that are connected with Tencent, Alipay, and WeChat. The person can enter his details, travel, and symptoms history. The three types of health codes are red, amber, and green. The person should follow the code he has been given. Red says that the person must be in quarantine for fourteen days, whereas amber indicates an individual must quarantine for seven days, and green indicates a person can go anywhere he wants. David Culver, CNN international correspondent, says his health QR code is green in Shanghai (Fig. **5**). Quick Response (QR) code permits modern smartphones to read universally and instantly recognize things. Japanese scientists first invented it in the year 1994. QR code removes friction and supports contactless capabilities in this COVID-19 outbreak. The tasks are completed effectively with zero wait time. It collects and stores a person's travel history easily and helps locate the contact people more quickly. Pandemic led to some other developments in China ZTE, a telecom provider, converted its conference room into 5G diagnosis systems.

Fig. (5). Health QR code shows green color, which implies that a scanned person is free to go anywhere.

Development of Drugs and Vaccines

Coronavirus is a worldwide hazard where the symptoms vary from cold to severe respiratory illnesses. The latest applications of AI are the virtual screening of new chemical entities. Network-based simulation is the primary approach to analyzing virus-host interactome. Benevolent AI of UK has applied AI-derived knowledge graphs to integrate biomedical data from structured and unstructured sources. Researchers at MIT and IBM have applied AI techniques to find antibiotics for COVID-19. Graph Convolutional Neural Networks (GCNN) are used in drug discovery applications. Machine Learning (ML) strategies such as SVM -Support Vector Machines, RF - Random Forest, and RFE - Recursive Feature Selection are essential tools to identify antigens from proteins. The research about drug discovery and vaccine are shared among scientists through IoT.

Technologies that emerged during the COVID-19 pandemic, such as Drone technology, robotics technologies, AI, and digital technologies, are given in Table 2.

Table 2. Emerging technologies used during the COVID-19 pandemic.

Technology	Application	Methodology	Organizations Developed such Technology
Robotics	Sanitation in hospitals	UV light robot	Xenex Disinfection Services
		Robot used for disinfectants	TMiRob
		UV-C disinfection robot	UVD Robots
		Cleaning robot	Seoul National University Hospital (SNUH)
	Sanitation in public places	Dispensing hand sanitizers	Zhen Robotics
	–	Robot for disinfection	Nanyang Technological University
	–	Robotic vacuum	SoftBank Robotics
	Patrolling	Robot for patrolling	Boston Dynamics
	–	Self-driving robot	Guangzhou Gosuncn Robot
	Screening	LIDAR and IR/optical cameras for screening	Ubtech
	–	Autonomous monitoring robots	Ubtech
	–	AI-powered, screening robot, videoconferencing	Robotemi

(Table 2) cont.....

Technology	Application	Methodology	Organizations Developed such Technology
AI technology	Healthcare consulting	Robots to give personal hygiene guidelines	SenseTime
	Assistance tool for a doctor	BotMD	National University Hospital Seng Hospital
	Monitoring public areas-screening	Scans 10 people per second	SenseTime
Digital Technology	Health care	5G technology	ZTE
	Tracking	Bluetooth based contact tracing	SGUnited
		GPS tracking and CCTV footage	South Korean government
		Digital QR health codes	Chinese government
	Daily life	Virtual Reality (VR)	Evergrande Sunshine Peninsula

CONCLUSION

COVID-19 is becoming a pandemic all over the world today. Scientists and researchers are trying to find out from where and how it emerged. On the other hand, all the developed and developing countries are working to create a vaccine and rapid testing facilities to control its spread. IoT is an emerging technology in various sectors, especially the healthcare system. IoT comes with personalized healthcare systems rather than conventional models. The chapter describes several technologies combined with IoT to fight against the COVID-19 pandemic. The technologies contribute to human society during the coronavirus outbreak in terms of symptom diagnosis, contact tracing, quarantine monitoring, and social distancing. Various applications designed using artificial intelligence in combination with IoT have been discussed.

ACKNOWLEDGEMENTS

The two authors have contributed ideas related to the world's threats faces due to COVID-19. Both authors contributed equally to the preparation of materials and data collection processes. All the authors have read the final manuscript and given approval.

REFERENCES

[1]   K. Ashton, "That internet of things", *RFiD.*, vol. 22, pp. 97-114, 2009.

[2]   G. Yang, L. Xie, M. Mantysalo, X. Zhou, Z. Pang, L.D. Xu, S. Kao-Walter, Q. Chen, and L.R. Zheng, "A health-IoT platform based on the integration of intelligent packaging, unobtrusive bio-sensor, and intelligent medicine box", *IEEE Trans. Industr. Inform.*, vol. 10, no. 4, pp. 2180-2191, 2014.
[http://dx.doi.org/10.1109/TII.2014.2307795]

[3]   J. Liu, X. Liao, S. Qian, J. Yuan, F. Wang, Y. Liu, Z. Wang, F.S. Wang, L. Liu, and Z. Zhang, "Community transmission of severe acute respiratory syndrome coronavirus 2, shenzhen, China, 2020", *Emerg. Infect. Dis.,* vol. 26, no. 6, pp. 1320-1323, 2020.
[http://dx.doi.org/10.3201/eid2606.200239] [PMID: 32125269]

[4]   T.G. Heck, R.Z. Frantz, M.N. Frizzo, C.H.R. François, M.S. Ludwig, M.A. Mesenburg, G.P. Buratti, L.B.B. Franz, and E.M. Berlezi, "Insufficient social distancing may contribute to COVID-19 outbreak: The case of Ijuí city in Brazil", *PLoS One,* vol. 16, no. 2, p. e0246520, 2021.
[http://dx.doi.org/10.1371/journal.pone.0246520] [PMID: 33596229]

[5]   N. Chen, M. Zhou, X. Dong, J. Qu, F. Gong, Y. Han, Y. Qiu, J. Wang, Y. Liu, Y. Wei, J. Xia, T. Yu, X. Zhang, and L. Zhang, "Epidemiological and clinical characteristics of 99 cases of 2019 novel coronavirus pneumonia in Wuhan, China: a descriptive study", *Lancet,* vol. 395, no. 10223, pp. 507-513, 2020.
[http://dx.doi.org/10.1016/S0140-6736(20)30211-7] [PMID: 32007143]

[6]   D.S. Hui, E. I Azhar, T.A. Madani, F. Ntoumi, R. Kock, O. Dar, G. Ippolito, T.D. Mchugh, Z.A. Memish, C. Drosten, A. Zumla, and E. Petersen, "The continuing 2019-nCoV epidemic threat of novel coronaviruses to global health — The latest 2019 novel coronavirus outbreak in Wuhan, China", *Int. J. Infect. Dis.,* vol. 91, pp. 264-266, 2020.
[http://dx.doi.org/10.1016/j.ijid.2020.01.009] [PMID: 31953166]

[7]   Y. Dong, and Y.D. Yao, "IoT Platform for COVID-19 Prevention and Control: A Survey", *IEEE Access,* vol. 9, pp. 49929-49941, 2021.
[http://dx.doi.org/10.1109/ACCESS.2021.3068276] [PMID: 34812390]

[8]   F. Bonomi, R. Milito, J. Zhu, and S. Addepalli, ''Fog computing and its role in the Internet of Things,'' in Proc. 1st Ed. MCC Workshop Mobile Cloud Comput. MCC, 2012, pp. 13–16.
[http://dx.doi.org/10.1145/2342509.2342513]

[9]   S.M. Kissler, C. Tedijanto, E. Goldstein, Y.H. Grad, and M. Lipsitch, "Projecting the transmission dynamics of SARS-CoV-2 through the postpandemic period", *Science,* vol. 368, no. 6493, pp. 860-868, 2020.
[http://dx.doi.org/10.1126/science.abb5793] [PMID: 32291278]

[10]   M.S. Rahman, N.C. Peeri, N. Shrestha, R. Zaki, U. Haque, and S.H.A. Hamid, "Defending against the Novel Coronavirus (COVID-19) outbreak: How can the Internet of Things (IoT) help to save the world?", *Health Policy Technol.,* vol. 9, no. 2, pp. 136-138, 2020.
[http://dx.doi.org/10.1016/j.hlpt.2020.04.005] [PMID: 32322475]

[11]   M. Nasajpour, S. Pouriyeh, R.M. Parizi, M. Dorodchi, M. Valero, and H.R. Arabnia, "Internet of things for current COVID-19 and future pandemics: an exploratory study", *J. Healthc. Inform. Res.,* vol. 4, no. 4, pp. 325-364, 2020.
[http://dx.doi.org/10.1007/s41666-020-00080-6] [PMID: 33204938]

[12]   A. Nayyar, B.L. Nguyen, and N.G. Nguyen, "The internet of drone things (IoDT): future envision of smart drones", *First International Conference on Sustainable Technologies for Computational Intelligence,* pp. 563-580 2020.
[http://dx.doi.org/10.1007/978-981-15-0029-9_45]

CHAPTER 4

Potential Applications of AI and IoT Collaborative Framework for Health Care

Lija Jacob[1,*], **K.T. Thomas**[1] and **Samiksha Shukla**[1]

[1] *Department of Data Science, CHRIST (Deemed to be University), Pune Lavasa Campus - The Hub of Analytics, Maharashtra 412112, India*

Abstract: Digital technology has infiltrated the entire planet. Artificial Intelligence (AI) and the Internet of Things (IoT) are the two buzzwords that became popular in the current digital world, especially in recent decades. Both these technologies have their contribution in various domains. The existing frameworks will benefit from the AI-IoT collaborative system, which will assist them in having more intelligent or smart responses. Furthermore, these collaborative systems can provide improved devices with better decision-making capacity to facilitate the users. AI can work with IoT to increase functional precision in the healthcare domain by automating and tracking, monitoring, managing, optimizing, and predicting processes in 24x7 mode. Health professionals are the people involved in activities whose primary commitment is to improve the wellbeing of the community. They are a group of people who face various obstacles, including their health and safety concerns, especially during pandemic outbreaks. This book chapter aims to illustrate the impact of AI and IoT on the health care domain and the challenges that healthcare professionals face, especially when dealing with such an pandemic and suggests some potential health care advancements through AI and IoT.

Keywords: Addiction Management, Artificial Intelligence, AI-IoT Collaborative Framework, AI-IoT Convergence, Community Units,, Cybersecurity, Disease Management, Electronic Health Record (EHR), Pandemic Outbreaks, HealthCare, Healthcare Workers, InClinic Segment, Intelligent Drones, Internet of Things, Internet of Medical Things (IoMT), In-home Segment, On-Body Device Units, Personal Emergency Response Systems (PERS), Smartphone Applications, Smart Wearables, Smart Kiosk, Telemedicine.

INTRODUCTION

The majority of healthcare practices are encounter-based, which means they are focused on the treatment of illness rather than its prevention.

---

[*] **Corresponding Author Lija Jacob:** Department of Data Science, CHRIST (Deemed to be University), Pune Lavasa Campus - The Hub of Analytics, Maharashtra 412112, India; Tel: +91 94474 73770; E-mail: lija.jacob@christuniversity.in

S. Vijayalakshmi, Naveen Chilamkurti, Savita, Rajesh Kumar Dhanaraj and Balamurugan Balusamy (Eds.)

As the population grows, there is a need for Artificial Intelligence (AI) based solutions to fasten the examination process and quickly provide the required medicine.

Digital transformation is bringing forth newtools and techniques to ease individuals' life. With the latest research and development in AI and the Internet of Things (IoT), this transformation is happening. The rise in new diseases led to an increase in healthcare expenses worldwide. There are various avenues in healthcare where AI can help and improve the medical facility. AI will help automate the process to provide context-specific information, analysis, and recommendations to patients, their relatives, and caregivers.

Many AI-based health services include identifying tumors, improving decision-making by looking into the previous data set, remote monitoring, and associated care.

The main concern in adopting the AI-based healthcare system is the ethical concern to be followed during the data collection and treatment period. On the one hand, patients are concerned about the privacy and confidentiality of individual data. On the other hand, practitioners face challenges as they need to equip themselves with new tools and technology. Technology is a blessing; at the same time, it may become a nightmare if not utilized correctly; it can harm the patient's life and the caregiver. Conclusion: many collaborative AI models offer better treatment and unprecedented opportunities to improve patient care and treatment outcomes. With the invention of AI-based medical care, patients, family members, and healthcare providers can get the recommendation and visualization of the information for collective decision-making.

There are many healthcare applications where AI is used, but it is crucial to adapt them with caution, or else we may end up with the user's disappointment. It is essential to involve various stakeholders in the development phase. Along with AI, IoT also plays a crucial role in healthcare systems to deliver high-quality services at a low cost. It is used for data collection, tracking, monitoring, identification, and authentication. Exponential growth has been observed in the field of IoT in healthcare [1].

This chapter discusses the various AI and IoT aspects. Section II & III present applications and frameworks available for healthcare professionals. Section IV explains some of the major contributions of AI in the field of healthcare. Section V presents smart health using AI and IoT. Section VI talks about the IoMT and its contribution to pandemic outbreaks.

AI IN HEALTHCARE

AI and other advancements in digital technology are playing a significant role in the community. AI growth is taking over many traditional models of healthcare. Patient care is taking a new dimension through AI in clinical analysis, surgery, and medicines. There are various types of research suggesting AI as a precision model in health care services. It is an opportunity as identifying disease in an early stage can help us in treatment before it becomes incurable [2].

Robots are leading the surgery, algorithms beating the pathologists and radiologists to identify harmful tumors in the initial stage. They are acting as a guide to physicians and other healthcare service providers. Although technology advancements are taking place, it is not easy to get acceptance, as there are incidences where patients prefer experience over technology. AI is helping in many fields to ease life, and healthcare is one among them. Fig. (1) shows the functions of AI in the healthcare domain.

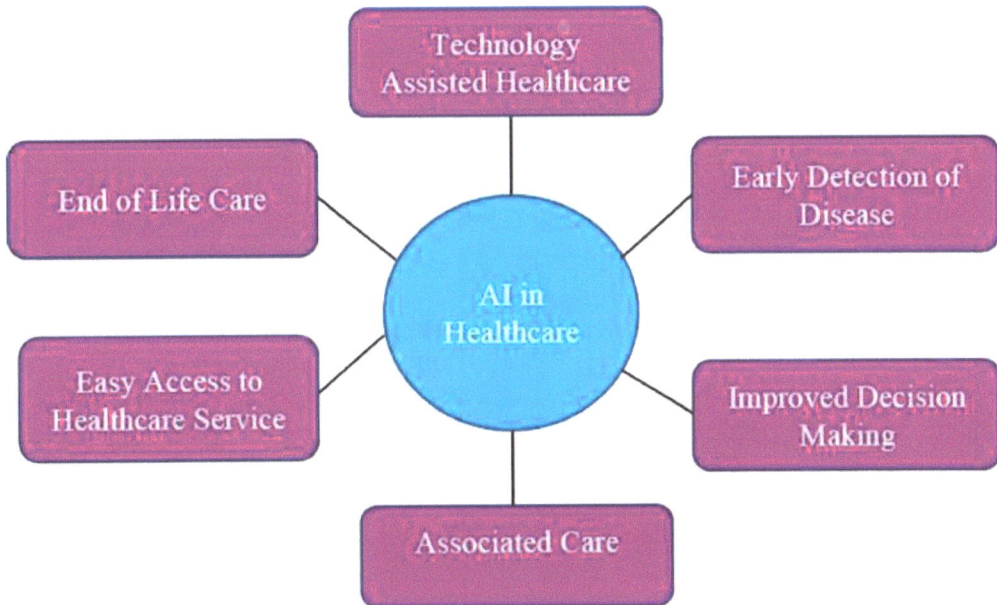

Fig. (1). Functions of AI in Healthcare.

Early Detection of Disease

AI is widely used in the early identification of diseases, such as tumors, and infections. According to the research, the sooner the disease is identified, the better is the treatment. The identification at an early stage leads to better treatment with less risk to life. AI-based techniques are faster and better than the other traditional techniques. With the help of wearable devices, it is easy to foresee health complications and act accordingly.

Improved Decision Making

The inclusion of AI in healthcare is a blessing for healthcare service providers and patients as well. The Electronic Health Record (EHR) of an individual's medical history and insightful assessment through the AI techniques help better decision-making. The EHR can assist caregivers and medical practitioners in promptly determining patients at risk and taking immediate actions.

Associated Care

The associated care is an essential element of any medical treatment. The medical treatment doesn't mean only the treatment by the doctors. To effectively and efficiently run the complete healthcare system, it requires many other people such as nurses, technicians, hospital management staff, pharmacists, *etc*.

Involvement of AI and IoT framework/techniques will help the caregivers and assist in alerting them immediately so the necessary action can be taken to identify the patients at risk of health declination.

Easy Access to Healthcare Services

With the support of the Electronic Health Records, AI and IoT frameworks assist those at high risk of heart stroke. AI can help medical practitioners by suggesting better treatment options for these patients. With the invention of robotic surgery, the expertise of doctors sitting miles away from the patient can be facilitated. The AI-based solution for the insurance industry helps patients by decreasing the hold-up times and reducing the staff's administrative workload. The modern healthcare systems based on AI and IoT can help us provide better treatment at ease. It reduces the requirement of qualified clinical staff to help individuals get the treatment as quickly as possible.

End of Life Care

Every living being has a life cycle; our body's strength and functions gradually decline towards the end of life. This capitulation of the body is generally due to cardiovascular breakdown, dementia, Cerebrovascular Disease, Diabetes, Porosis, *etc*. AI-enabled robots can help with the end-of-life care; they can facilitate the aged people to remain self-ruling to reduce hospitalization and provide facilities at home. It has the potential to improve the end-of-life experience for senior citizens and others suffering from life-threatening illnesses.

Technology-Assisted Healthcare

These days due to advancements in technology assisted healthcare is on the hike. The IoT is helping to develop a smart home solution for various state-of-the-art products and services. This IoT-based solution can assist older people by providing telemedicine facilities, social connections, and activities to engage the individual, location-based services to make them move freely. These technologies are used for personalized medicines, health monitoring, smart drugs, and health-as- a-service (HaaS). Technology-Assisted healthcare acts as a blessing for those who need critical care; with these techniques, health monitoring can be done with ease at home comfort.

Challenges in AI and IoT Based Healthcare System

There are many global health challenges faced while using AI and IoT-enabled healthcare services. The healthcare system involves many people, including hospital staff, nurses, doctors, pharmacists, institutions, and resources. The health care framework is not based on simple automation-based pre-defined rules, but it is based on continuous learning, absorption, and decision-making based on AI and IoT frameworks. This learning is based on the constant monitoring of users' habits and behavior in the intelligent environment. This comfort and ease come with many challenges related to learning new technology and upgrading themselves in case of any advancement in the technology. Sometimes these methods lack precision, fault tolerance, and stability.

The adoption of technology brings about privacy and security challenges. These IoT devices are prone to security attacks. The integrity of many of these IoT devices is the biggest challenge, they cannot be interconnected, or unique integration solutions are required if connected. There are many challenges such as Physical and Operational Challenges such as the availability of technicians to operate the high- end devices. The costs of the devices are too high which is a barrier for many healthcare service providers to install such devices. The healthcare system involves many stakeholders so getting their consent and bringing them in the process is the biggest challenge. Although we have many advantages of adapting AI and IoT-driven healthcare facilities, bringing these technologies into the workforce is challenging too.

AI-IOT COLLABORATIVE FRAMEWORK

The current tech world of analytics is trending unquestionably more into the world of cloud and computing. Two of the most remarkable innovations in technology were IoT and AI. The network of smart devices, sensors, or any physical objects that can actively communicate and have the computing capability to generate, exchange, and utilize data with nominal human involvement is the Internet of Things (IoT) [3]. Artificial intelligence or AI denotes the mockup of human intelligence using machines trained to think or act like humans [4]. Artificial intelligence is supported by any equipment that exhibits behaviors associated with a human mind, such as learning and problem-solving. When both robust technologies are unified, the world will be led to a nifty tech future. The combination of the technologies has revolutionized transformation in the industrial domain, including robotics, automation and engineering, and smart appliances in their production.

The integration of IoT with AI created more intelligent, innovative, and accurate machines and products with the competence to link through methodological and technical inheritance without human interference. The amount of data generated using the network of devices, sensors, and users is enormous. AI methodologies assist in gaining knowledge and developing intelligent applications or smarter products. The applications or products ease the improvement and progression in various domains, which are limited to education, healthcare, communal security, conveyance, and energy sectors. The success of today's IoT-based digital economy depends heavily on artificial intelligence [5].

IoT-powered artificial intelligence can produce intelligent products. However, this process needs to comply with security requirements in computation, transmission, resource usage, and efficiency at the same time. Fig. (**2**) depicts the AI-IoT Framework.

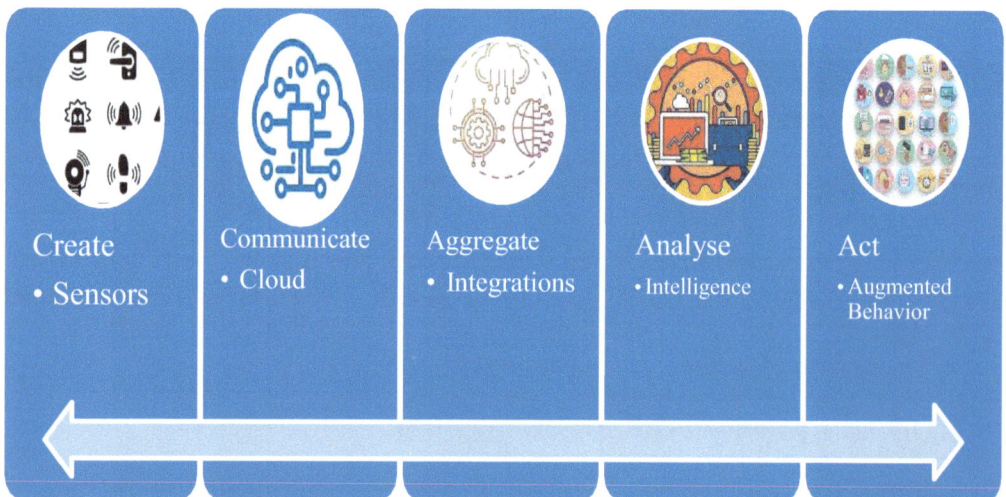

Fig. (2). AI-IoT framework.

Transformation of IoT with AI

The Internet of Things is centered on sensors implanted into machines, which collect information *via* Internet connectivity. To succeed, every IoT-related service must follow five basic steps: Create, Communicate, Aggregate, Analyze, and Act [6]. A crucial aspect of the "Act" is its penultimate analysis. This means that IoT is excellently assessed at its analysis stage. Here, artificial intelligence plays an essential role.

Benefits of AI-IoT Integration

AI and IoT together make a powerful combination. AI technology can act as a key to unlock IoT potential. Together, they are referred to as AIoT. AI can extract insights quickly from data in this context, which is its value. AI technology based on machine learning allows categorizing the patterns and detecting glitches in the data generated by smart sensors and devices-information such as temperatures, pressures, moisture, air quality, atmospheres and sounds. Machine learning approaches can produce effective predictions up to 20 times faster and that with more accuracy than outmoded business analytical tools. These methods frequently keep an eye out for numerical thresholds that need to be crossed. Speech recognition, computer vision, and other AI technologies can help gain insight into data once requiring human analysis [7].

The following are some benefits of integrating AI and IoT:

a. Increased working efficiency and productivity- Companies that employ AI in IoT applications can enhance their productivity. AI is capable of handling information and making forecasts in a way that people cannot. A short period can be used to accomplish an enormous amount of information. Integrating AI and IoT will not only benefit the employer; it will also help customers. It can also personalize a customer's experience if the strategy is executed correctly.

b. Building new and improved products-By integrating AI into IoT, new products and services can also be created. Shortly, natural language processing (NLP) will allow people to communicate with machines without a human operator. The introduction of AI-controlled drones and robots that can travel where humans cannot bring up new monitoring and inspection possibilities.

c. Enhancement of Security and Safety-Integrating AI and IoT can allow for an enhanced degree of security if they are done effectively.

d. Improved risk management-In addition to automating rapid reactions, IoT and AI applications can help organizations improve worker security, monetary loss and cyber incidents. This can be achieved through programs that can detect fraudulent behavior at bank ATMs; or predictions based on the driving patterns for identifying auto insurance premiums; Identifying the dangerous conditions for factory workers with the help of a surveillance program, and surveillance by law enforcement to identify prospective crime scenes in advance.

AI-IoT Convergence: Real-world Use Cases

The mutually advantageous rapport between the Artificial Intelligence (AI) and the Internet of Things (IoT) empowered the development of disruptive novelties in innumerable domains. It comes in various forms like wearables, embedded, biomedical devices which can be used for health care monitoring or autonomous drones for smart surveillance, devastation administration, relief operations management and rescue operations.

This section gives us a glimpse of various domains where the fusion of AI and IOT has proven the track of records with more predictive and autonomous products where even a large amount of data has to be handled. The collection of large amounts of data is driven with the help of IoT devices, where at the same time, AI will support deriving the intelligence for formulating smarter products for the smarter space. In addition, the evolution of 5G technology will pave the way to reveal the wide-ranging potential of AI-driven IoT in varied realms. In this current world, many industries have designed and created business models incorporating the concepts of AI-controlled IoT. The following are a few examples.

Autonomous Driving

IoT, as well as AI, becomes more evident with self-directed driving. The sensors constantly gather data about the environment or surrounding through continuous measurements. The data collected using the sensors is processed in the Autonomous/Self-driving vehicles, and intelligent decision-making and insights are developed with the help of AI models implemented in it. Thus, the real-time navigation system enables the vehicle to negotiate to surround and plan complex routes in real-time.

Using AI, a self-driving car can predict road conditions, optimal speed, weather, pedestrian behavior, *etc.* They can also become progressively smarter as they travel.

AI-driven Robots

With implanted sensors, robots in factories are becoming more intelligent, which facilitates data transmission. Additionally, since robots have artificial intelligence algorithms, they can learn from continually updated data. This approach significantly reduces downtime and potentially saves money, and thus simplifying the overall production process.

Embedding AI in Cybersecurity

AI-powered cybersecurity systems can distinguish network breaches, thereby protecting valuable data and stopping cyber-attacks.

AI-powered systems can learn how to identify standard activity patterns and spot anomalous activity, thereby reducing false alerts and detecting potential cyber-attacks.

Artificial Intelligence (AI)-based Smart Appliances

With advances in artificial intelligence, technology has evolved to meaningful collaboration between humans and machines. Additionally, virtual assistants, also known as digital assistants, use voice-controlled artificial intelligence to perform functions such as searching the internet, making phone calls, and connecting to other devices. A smartphone can contain one of these devices or be used as a standalone device. It is an excellent way to make home appliances work more effectively and efficiently.

Following is a list of possible scenarios for utilizing AI in appliances:

Smart Speakers

A smart speaker is the most trending device that utilizes artificial intelligence and machine learning. In terms of technology, any speaker that can perform any activity other than music can be called a smart speaker. Voice commands can control smart speakers, such as creating a playlist, setting reminders, making grocery lists, and even searching the internet.

Smart Laundry Machines

A smart washer can automatically adjust its washing strength and detergent according to the load weight and the type of fabric by utilizing AI techniques. An alert can also be sent automatically if there is no detergent in stock. Studies have revealed that adopting such technologies enables users to reduce detergent consumption by 30% and save energy and resources.

Intelligent Refrigerators

Deep learning is used in Intelligent Refrigerators to monitor and recognize food in the refrigerator remotely. A refrigerator inventory list can automatically be created from all the information, making it easy for anyone to keep track of what's inside. The application will also let the user select an item from the fridge and view relevant recipes suitable for that item. Users can also upload photos to smart fridges to create shopping lists, check inside the refrigerator to see what items are out of stock and create shopping lists using smartphones. It is possible to monitor the fridge and freezer's temperature as well.

AI-IOT CONTRIBUTION IN THE HEALTHCARE DOMAIN

The healthcare industry or medical industry provides products and services within an economic system that treat, prevent, rehabilitate, and provide palliative or end-of-life care. A modern health care system consists of various sub-sections. Individuals' and populations' health needs are met by interdisciplinary teams of skilled professionals and paraprofessionals. AI-IoT convergence was a big boon for various domains and has proved helpful in healthcare. The usage of the Internet of Things (IoT) in the realms of health care, especially in the industry and applications, has drastically increased.

As AI-IoT surged in popularity, its contributions to healthcare gained more attention, with improvements in diagnostic accuracy, remote monitoring, telemedicine, reduced waiting times, automated recording, updating, and maintenance of records and assets

With our technological boom in AI and IoT, the scope of telemedicine was further broadened. In the healthcare industry, AI and IoT together can save lives with the most effective and time-efficient mechanisms, like Smart Medicare, home health care systems, real-time health monitoring, and emergency alarm systems. Hence the AI-IoT collaborative framework can be called 'life-saving technology".

It is becoming increasingly evident that smart medical sensors and IoT devices are drastically reshaping the healthcare industry in the worldwide scenario to a more automated model. The impact has grown due to the proven performance of real-time applications support.

Smart medical sensors and Internet-of-things devices have been developing rapidly in recent times, and these devices are profoundly changing the way healthcare is provided worldwide. The Cloud and IoT architectures, combined with AI technology, have covered the way for the development of Intelligent healthcare technologies that are capable of processing and performing intelligence on the significant amount of data generated by wearable sensor networks in real-time.

The following diagram in Fig. (**3**) shows the different applications of AI in healthcare from various perspectives. Some of the use cases where collaboration between AI and IoT has contributed to the healthcare industry. Let us discuss some of the use cases where AI-IoT is contributing to the healthcare domain.

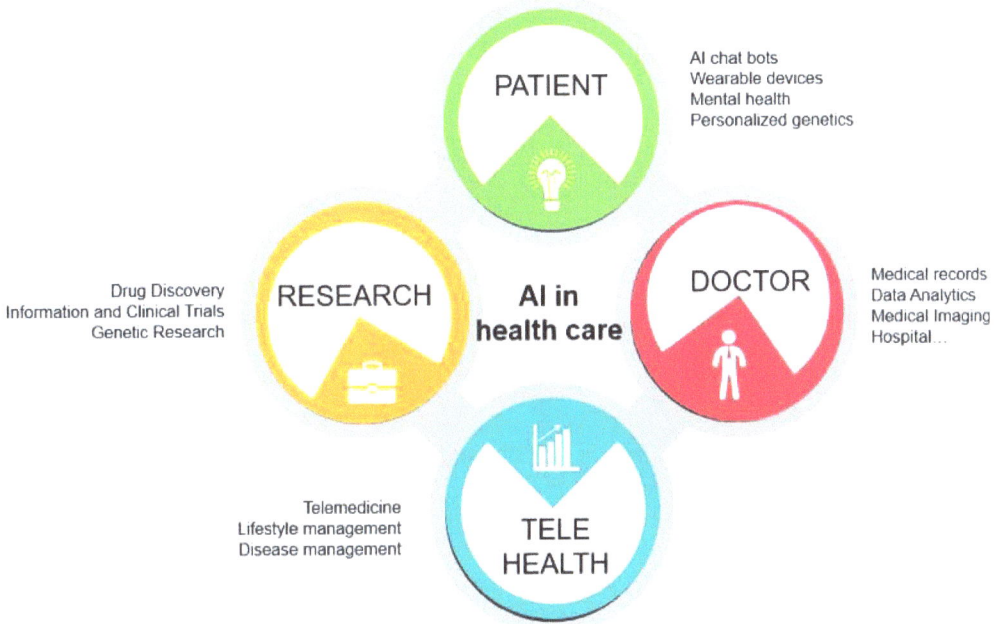

Fig. (3). Different Applications of AI in healthcare.

Patient Tracking and Predicting Staffing Requirements

It is natural for hospitals to generate vast amounts of data. Patient information such as Heart rate, blood pressure, temperature, and even the visual data like x-rays and CT scans of the patient can be invaluable for determining the best treatment at the right time [8]. With the new technology such as AI and the Internet of Things (IoT), this information can be made accessible to doctors . Thus, AI-IoT Integrated technology is transforming hospitals where they are applied. Let us see how this has become practical in the real-time hospital scenario.

Patient data through the usage of Wearable Devices- It is critical to collect vital readings on patients on a regular basis in order to deliver the right drugs. Readings include temperatures, heartbeats, blood pressure, oxygen concentration in the blood, and blood sugar levels. Health professionals may need to revisit these patients periodically and be physically present with them to measure these symptoms. This increases the risk of infection in patients.

Wearable devices that can measure all vitals from patients at a set time are an important application of the Internet of Things in healthcare. The wearable device will collect all of the data with the help of various sensors and transfer it to the IoT Gateway for processing *via* Bluetooth, ZigBee, or other wireless protocols. Data from the cloud can be collected and analyzed by providers for necessary decisions. A nursing station is notified immediately by the system when a patient is in critical condition. An alarm is triggered when the temperature increases or oxygen levels fall from certain levels.

Fitbits, activity trackers, and wearables are increasingly being adopted by health-conscious individuals themselves to manage their health proactively. Wearable fitness devices like fit bits track physical activity, sleep patterns, hydration levels, electrocardiograms, and body temperatures. These devices enable patients and doctors to exchange information, leading to better treatment and lower overall costs and allowing them to detect changes in patient conditions earlier than they would otherwise be able to do.

Embedding AI and ML algorithms in these systems not only helps identify and prioritize high-risk groups but also helps navigate and monitor data from the devices that patients use to guide treatment protocols.

Wearables powered by artificial intelligence can be great aids for healthcare providers because they improve mobility, autonomy, accuracy, and ease of use.

Predicting staffing requirements-Soon, artificial intelligence algorithms can analyze patient electronic health records and predict what staffing requirements will be necessary to manage the risk posed by the patient. Typically, hospitals can meet these requirements well with contingent workforce hiring.

Diagnostics *via* Telemedicine or Remote Diagnosis

During the lockdown and the pandemic, hospitals are not easily accessible, making regular checkups and medical care impossible. Telemedicine and remote diagnostics are highly beneficial during this time, as many patients avoid travel. A teleconsultation is an opportunity to conduct a virtual visit without exposing staff to direct contact with patients.

The doctor may make a diagnosis and write prescriptions for the patient *via* a variety of communication methods, including video, audio, text, and data exchange. Critical patient information may not always be accurately delivered through these communication channels. However, a portable IoT device enables different data to be collected and sent to the doctor to prescribe the proper medication. These devices can collect relevant and precise data, such as body temperature, blood sugar levels, and blood oxygen levels, from a distance., as well as digital images of the ears, throat, and other parts of the patient's body.

More than half of all human deaths are caused by chronic diseases like diabetes, cardiovascular disorders, and cancer. A new technique for treating chronic diseases includes devices like sensors, facts, and algorithms, as well as medical professionals. The framework mainly consists primarily of four functionalities:

a. Gather physiological data in the hospital and at home;

b. Data from several sources is combined to create a full picture of a patient's health

c. Recognize the signs and symptoms of a chronic illness.

d. Monitor the progress of the disease and help the patient manage it.

Disease Management in Chronic Illness

CDM (Chronic Disease Management) is a comprehensive approach to managing chronic diseases or other conditions that are long-lasting in their effects. According

to the studies, 50 percent of individuals suffer from asthma, arthritis, diabetes, heart disease, and chronic obstructive pulmonary disease (COPD). Diabetes and heart disease are the two most expensive and common chronic diseases. Diabetes and heart disease are the two most expensive and common chronic diseases [9].

In addition to high healthcare costs, screenings, checkups, monitoring and coordinating treatment, and patient education, are some of the most significant challenges in managing chronic disease. While clinician judgment cannot be replaced, new data-driven technologies, including AI, can improve patient care by ensuring the proper care is given at the right time.

Using AI in combination with IoT for complete healthcare digitization can enable patients to get proactive disease treatment and preventive care, drawing actionable conclusion from their data.

Addiction Management

Another revolution in the healthcare domain with the AI-IoT framework is addiction management. Let's look at some of the ways IoT and AI can treat addiction.

The Habit Tracker

AI programs with IoT products can track many of our habits, which is quite remarkable. Monitoring and individual addiction can be done creatively by using sensor networks. QuitBit is an application that analyzes smoking habits. It examines, for example, when and on which days they smoke. Cloud-based AI-IoT systems can record smoking patterns and predict when users will smoke. In response, the user will receive an encouraging message encouraging them to delay smoking for a while or to suggest playing a game or taking a walk instead.AI algorithms aim to treat smoking addiction through distractions and a points system actively. Such engaging approaches like these can be more effective in overcoming addictive habits.

The AI-IoT Breath Analyzer

There is a great deal of potential for AI and IoT developments to prevent addicts from harm. A breathalyzer that uses AI and IoT can detect the breath to detect alcohol consumption to determine how often and what amount of alcohol is consumed. As we have seen, IoT and artificial intelligence can have many benefits for addiction treatment.

Reduced Waiting Times in Emergency Rooms (ER); Fastest Attention to Critical Patients and Handling Shortages of Doctors

AI is enabling hospitals to reduce the shortage of doctors and patient waiting times. Artificial intelligence-enabled systems and automatic bed-tracking systems alert hospital staff when an empty bed is available, helping them admit emergency patients more quickly and reducing their admission wait time. With hospitals at capacity and overburdened, it is more essential than ever to identify patients who need urgent attention. The process is difficult. Nurses and doctors must make snap decisions under colossal pressure and analyze a lot of data. AI-enhanced virtual assistants can help hospitals rescue the sickest patients. Doctors are alerted when a patient's condition worsens in these systems, and their vitals are analyzed. AI hospital systems were sometimes able to spot problems missed by doctors. In turn, this would result in a significant reduction in mortality rates. Artificial Intelligence is an "effective tool" used to mine data to help diagnose and manage diseases similar to how physicians diagnose them.

Thus, investing in technologically driven approaches to healthcare can avoid long wait times for medical services and doctor shortages [10].

Automated Robotic Processes

Robotics and automation make hospital activities such as delivering medications to patients and performing complex surgeries easier. Inpatients can gain access to medicine, food, and other essentials from robotic carts, reducing the need for close human contact. Additionally, robotics and automation allow medical staff to serve more patients as mundane tasks are done by the robots instead of the staff. Moreover, robotic assistants can also collect and automatically enter a variety of patient information into their Electronic Health Records (EHR) through various sensors. This data can be used for a variety of purposes, including assessing whether medications are taken by patients when given by cart and monitoring and updating patient vital statistics using an AI-enabled camera. AR-VR technology allows surgeons to operate remotely with high precision while performing complex surgeries.

Air purifiers with intelligence, such as Smart Air Purifiers, ensure clean air and great air quality. When the air quality index declines, connected air purifiers notify the hospital, and all purifiers can be operated remotely *via* a dashboard and a mobile application. Automatic disinfectants with robots are used to clean hospital spaces, operating theatres, and contaminated patient rooms. As a result, human intervention should be decreased, and virus propagation can be controlled.

AI-IoT for COVID-19

Keeping an appropriate distance between crowds is vital during pandemic situations, especially when crowds gather, such as the patient ward, the laboratories, and pharmacy areas, because such crowding may contribute to disease spread. As a result, in order to maintain social division, people must be controlled in certain regions. Using wearable devices with geo-tracking sensors, wearers can receive updates regarding their current location and receive notifications when they exceed predetermined boundaries at specific locations. The administrator can use information from gadgets to deliver announcements to clear the space and maintain social distance, through a paging system.

Mass Screening in Pandemic

A mass screening campaign has been suggested as a preventative measure to keep the disease from spreading. The use of wearable devices equipped with IoT sensors can also monitor conditions throughout certain regions. Mass populations data can be collected at a central location or *via* cloud services, such as mass temperature screening. These gadgets record the temperature readings and communicate them to the cloud on a regular basis. This large volume of data can be analyzed by Artificial Intelligence combining Machine Learning algorithms to provide statistics in which city temperatures are rising as more people flock to the city. Health authorities can identify and trace infected individuals' Bluetooth-enabled wearable devices.

Following are other possible use cases during a COVID-19 Pandemic:

a. Devices equipped with Bluetooth also alert users when they do not maintain social distances in public places. If a Bluetooth device is within six feet of another device, it'll vibrate or emit a beep if the distance is less than six feet. In addition, it alerts the user if infected people have come within 6 feet of him.

b. Authorities cannot trace a person without knowing their current location in real-time. Using a wearable device is helpful for travelers who need to enter quarantine during travel from another country or city. If a person exits the quarantine region during the duration of quarantine, the device's geolocation tracking alerts the authorities.

c. The COVID-19 virus, according to researchers, enters the human body by the eyes, nose, or mouth. Artificial Intelligence devices can also detect and notify users by touching their faces, noses, or eyes by utilizing proximity sensors. It comes in handy when you plan to use the device outdoors in a public place.

d. During the pandemic, AI-IoT drones have been popular for a variety of activities, including disinfectant spraying, monitoring affected regions, and transporting commodities. In the post-COVID-19 era, drones could be instrumental in sanitizing outer areas of the hospital, large compounds, and so on. It facilitates the delivery of medicines to zones infected with disease, thereby alleviating medical staff burdens. Furthermore, the usage of drones speeds up the process of blood, vaccine, and emergency injection supplies.

e. Drones can conduct remote monitoring of infected areas and hospitals. Its AI-enabled camera can identify anomalies in this area and help ambulances clear traffic on their routes with their connected cameras. As a result, a cloud platform receives various data from connected drones equipped with IoT sensors for further analysis and decision making.

SMART HEALTH USING AI AND IOT

In a world of advanced sensory media, things, and cloud computing, "Smart Healthcare" has emerged as a trend receiving tremendous attention from universities, government, industry, and healthcare providers. Last few years we have witness the growth of the Internet of Things (IoT) which has brought more than a billion pieces of data into reality and many services. Almost every domain

adopts artificial intelligence (AI) algorithms for machine learning, even for highly complex areas such as patient care. In addition to being incredibly revolutionary, AI and IoT can both benefit from convergence. By enabling deeper insight into healthcare data to support cheap individualized care, AI-driven IoT can make a big contribution to smart healthcare. In addition, it can provide real-time decision-making and robust processing of large IoT data volumes (big data) at a scale that goes beyond the capability of individual "things."IoT-oriented artificial intelligence (AIIoT) for smart healthcare has the potential to change many aspects of our healthcare business; nevertheless, technical difficulties must be overcome before the full promise of AIIoT can be realized.; however, technical challenges remain before they can fully be tapped.

The following sections describe how AI-IoT has benefited the medical domain from a health care professional's or layperson's perspective.

Smartphone Applications Incorporating AI and IoT

Increasingly, hospitals are using mobile apps to improve the management of workflows and facilitate clinical communication between providers and patients. The use of mobile apps streamlines communication between patients, providers, and caregivers and allows 24X7 monitoring of a patient's condition with the ability to personalize healthcare.

Healthcare apps fall into the category of health and wellness. Both are very similar but have quite a few differences. Health apps are mobile applications that diagnose, track or treat diseases. A wellness app is a mobile application that monitors the user's overall health. Aside from addressing genuine health concerns, these apps can address social, economic, environmental, or spiritual issues that affect one's well-being.

Mobile healthcare app development has become an essential part of healthcare providers adapting to ever-changing patient needs and staying ahead of their competitors. By partnering with digital experts to build quality mobile experiences, health care providers will increase patient loyalty -- resulting in higher revenue in the present and the future.

The typical healthcare apps are not limited to functionalities like DNA & Nutrition, Online Counseling, Custom Acne Treatment, Diabetes Tracker Log, Eye Care Live, 24X7 Access to a Doctor.

Healthcare providers are increasingly relying on mobile apps to support their ability to grow and meet the rapidly evolving needs of their patients. Smartphone applications can be more effective if they can be used without human intervention and can aid in driving us to perfect decisions.

Fitness apps are examples of AI-based apps that connect users to a store of food and calorie information through IoT and offer proper diet advice; global positioning system (GPS) apps that track users' fitness progress.

A successful app ensures the following features:

User Friendly

It's essential to have health apps that enable patients to book, change, and cancel doctors' appointments efficiently. The best wellness apps provide patients with quick access to information, the ability to review data, and the option to share data with a healthcare provider. Through AI-IoT-based smart healthcare mobile apps, doctors can access patient data gathered when patients booked appointments. Consequently, the system helps to avoid the wastage of time taken for pre-examination at hospitals. The app can even make some predictions based on the data collected.

Data Accuracy and Accessibility

Healthcare applications need to provide clear, actionable information to users. Ideally, a smart healthcare app should ensure the accuracy of the readings taken by its devices. Additionally, it should be able to accommodate patients with disabilities. All users should be catered to and provided with valuable and helpful features. Consumers usually download apps for healthcare to learn more about their condition and causes and take action when necessary. Apps must provide interactive tools that engage users and make them feel that their care is individualized.

Easy Communication with Professionals

Studies have shown that most doctors, ERs, and urgent care visits can be handled *via* phone or video. The average time for an in-person visit was also calculated to be 121 minutes. Patients and practitioners can save a great deal of time using apps if they are appropriately designed. Telehealth services have to be able to provide the same or better experiences as face-to-face doctor-patient interaction.

Smart Wearables for Monitoring, Diagnosis, and Prediction

With the help of wearable devices, human physical activity and behaviors can be continuously monitored. The most common methods to assess vital signs are electrocardiograms (ECGs), ballistocardiograms (BCGs), and other measures such as blood pressure, temperature, and pulse rate. Additional clinical data can be gathered using a photo or video device. Accessories such as sunglasses, eyeglasses, ears, clothing, gloves, and watches can be worn with a wearable device. A wearable device may also evolve into a skin-attachable device. Sensors can be implanted in chairs, automobile seats, and mattresses. Smartphones, in most circumstances, capture data and send it to a distant server for storage and analysis.

AI-enabled technology can significantly increase the capability of today's wearable devices. Many AI-led technologies, including machine learning, gesture recognition, and more, are incorporated into these sophisticated algorithms. With high-value data, users experience a more personalized experience. Three broad factors are driving the growth of wearable AI:

• Improved wearable hardware

• Improved AI algorithms

• Improvement in wireless connectivity such as the advent of 5G

Smart Pulse Oximeter: The pulse rate, arterial oxygen saturation (SO2), respiration rate, and perfusion index of a person are all monitored with this gadget. The instrument determines how much oxygen and haemoglobin are present in the blood. The devices can be operated by placing them on one's fingertip or earlobe. They are useful in emergency situations, patients with respiratory or cardiac problems, and people who suffer from sleep disturbances. This technology is useful for pilots, mountain climbers, and sportsmen who need to monitor oxygen levels or physical activity at high altitudes.

Smart Watches: The watches can be used to make and receive calls and track fitness activities. They have long-lasting batteries. Exercises are shown on screens, calories burned and active minutes are reported, sleep patterns are monitored, heart rates are monitored, running distance is tracked, *etc*. The majority of big smartphone companies are producing these watches in order to capitalize on the growing sector.

Smart Contact Lenses: A Google-developed lens, these lenses help people with poor eyesight and diabetes. Their measurements are based on the glucose content of the tears of an individual. They assist in the restitution of the natural autofocus of the eye.

AI-based Personal Emergency Response Systems (AI-PERS)

A Personal Emergency Response System (PERS) is a sort of personal emergency response system that is also known as a Medical Emergency Response System (MERS). It can help people in times of emergency or simply in case of an emergency by surfacing when we need assistance. PERS systems usually consist of three components:

In a PERS, three components are installed: a small radio transmitter, a console hooked up to your phone and a center that monitors emergency calls [11].

The devices can be worn on wrist bands, belts, or in your pocket with lightweight battery-powered transmitters. Users can trigger the help button on the transmitter to signal the console when they need help. An emergency number is automatically called from the console. With PERS, seniors and other vulnerable individuals can live independently by providing reassurance and ongoing monitoring.

Considering the increased public and private involvement in elder care, the trend towards home healthcare, the longer average life expectancy, and the burgeoning baby boomer population, even a typical individual can benefit from PERS.

Some artificial intelligence-based PERS systems, such as Corti, use machine learning for life-saving diagnostic assistance. With artificial intelligence, such as Corti software, critical illnesses such as cardiac arrest can be diagnosed in real-time with speech recognition, language analysis, and sound and background noise analysis. Emergency dispatchers can diagnose situations faster and formulate response strategies more quickly.

Intelligent Drones

A drone is a machine that flies without human interaction. In general, it is used for remote monitoring. Drones are also called unmanned aircraft vehicles (UAVs) equipped with sensors, GPS, and communications services and are known as IoT-integrated drones. The Internet of Drone Things (IoDT) makes it possible for drones to do multiple things; it can provide additional value to users' various tasks, including searching, monitoring, and delivering [12].

With a smartphone and a controller, smart drones can be controlled with minimal effort and time, making them convenient for various uses, such as agriculture, training, the healthcare industry, and other missions.

AI-IoT-based drones used in healthcare include various types such as a thermal imaging drone, a disinfectant drone, a medical drone, a surveillance drone, an announcement drone, and a multipurpose drone.

In epidemiology, drones are used for research into disease spread and to monitor disaster sites and zones. There is a growing demand for telemedicine drones for diagnosis, perioperative evaluation, and telemonitoring in remote locations. The medical applications of drones include microbiology, lab testing, pharmaceuticals, vaccines, emergency medical equipment, and patient transportation.

There are three types of medical drone applications catastrophe relief/public health, telemedicine, and medical transportation. Disaster relief, mass casualty care, data collection, communicable disease, and critical care are just a few of the key fields that fall under the umbrella of public health/disaster relief.

In telemedicine, drones have been used to support surgical procedures in scenarios like the battlefield and as telemedical devices in emergencies. The medical products and transportation articles include deliveries of medical supplies, patient evacuations, and commercial infrastructure applications.

The significant applications of drones in healthcare can be summarized as shown in Fig. (**4**).

A drone can spread the medical supplies that patients require. At present, drones are used to distribute medical supplies, but at some point, smaller indoor drones might deliver medicines from the pharmacy to patients' bedsides.

The medication would then be administered more quickly and less likely to contain errors. Nursing and pharmacy staff can work more efficiently with supplies brought directly to the patient to gather item by item. As an alternative to hospital-based care, drones could deliver medications and supplies to patients at home. It is anticipated that both outpatient care and home-based care will become more prevalent in the future. Providing home-based care may be more accessible and safer with drone technology for many conditions. Providers can use drones to take blood from a patient at home and send it immediately to the lab for testing. The provider may use drones to deliver medications, antibiotics, and other treatments to the patients at home.

Smart Kiosks

AI Healthcare Kiosks are touchless diagnostic devices that use artificial intelligence to provide a holistic and complete view of a person's health and wellness. Using these multiple kiosks worldwide, these devices offer solutions that include triage, remote diagnosis, insurance automation, and second opinions. A patient's basic body parameters and measurements include their weight, height, BMI, blood pressure, pulse, temperature, as well as the completion of a diagnostic triage to determine whether an x-ray may be required. Some hospitals have developed extra modules for Novel coronavirus that include IR scans and chest x-ray analysis using convolutional neural networks in conjunction with custom enzymes designed from synthetic biology-based on Serology. The kiosk is designed to provide complete diagnostic solutions to the patient while they walk in. The emphasis would be on proactive rather than reactive treatment. The kiosk offers a facility for needle-free blood collection from the arm.

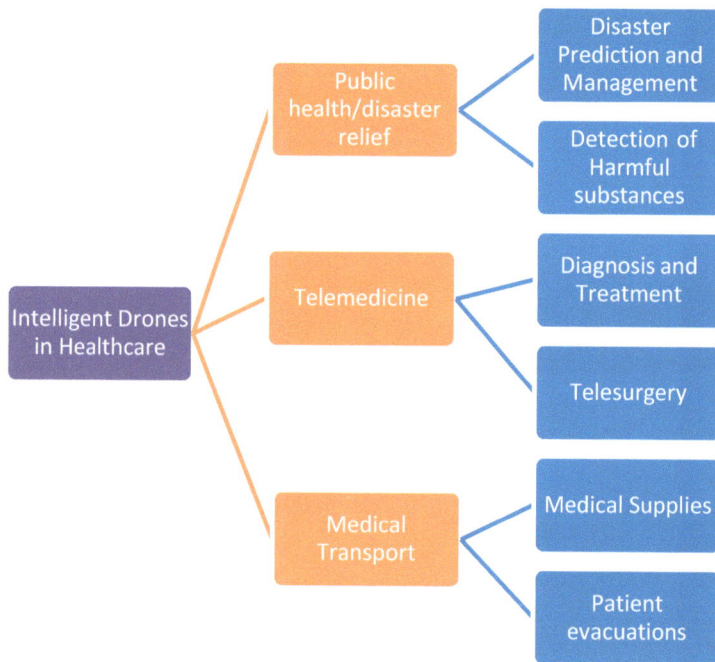

Fig. (4). Major applications of the drones.

INTERNET OF MEDICAL THINGS (IOMT) FOR PANDEMIC OUTBREAKS

The 'Internet of Medical Things (IoMT)' is a collection of devices and applications that are networked to health-care information systems [13]. It allows people to communicate with their doctors and securely transmit medical records, reducing unnecessarily frequent hospital visits, putting pressure on the health-care system.

A large part of the IoMT market consists of smart devices for health care applications, such as wearable devices and medical/vital monitors, either at home or in the field, and their associated services, such as telehealth and real-time location.

On-Body Device Units

Consumer and medical units can be found in on-body health wearables. Consumer health wearables include activity trackers, bracelets, wristbands, sports watches, and smart clothing, as well as consumer-level gadgets that enable wellness or fitness monitoring. Although these gadgets are not regulated centrally, experts may advocate them for certain health uses based on consumer studies and informal clinical validation [13].

Usually, clinical-grade wearables include regulated devices and supporting platforms that have been approved or certified by one or more regulatory or health agencies. Medical advice or a prescription is usually required to use these devices. Smarter belts, such as Active Protective, deploy hip protection when a wearer falls; headsets can improve muscle memory, strength, and endurance by stimulating brain areas necessary for exercise and physical training.

In-home Segment

There are three main segments of in-home healthcare: personal emergency response systems (PERS), remote patient monitoring (RPM), and telehealth virtual visits [13].

PERS is a composite method that integrates wearable electronics with a medical call centre to assist the elderly in becoming more self-reliant. The package can provide easy and fast access to emergency medical care.

Sensors and systems for remote home monitoring assist in the management of chronic illness by continuously monitoring physiological indicators to help avoid or control illness. They support long-term care in the patient's home by limiting the disease progression; enable acute home monitoring to aid patients' recovery and avoid rehospitalization; and medication management to provide reminders, and dosage information, and enhance medication adherence.

A virtual telehealth appointment can help people manage their health conditions and acquire prescriptions or treatment recommendations. Video consultations, video monitoring, and digital tests to assess symptoms or lesions are some of these options.

Community Units

The community segment has five components [13]:

a. Mobility Services: During transit, health parameters can be tracked by vehicles with mobility services.

b. Emergency response intelligence: - During an emergency, emergency response intelligence assists first responders, paramedics, and hospital emergency department staff.

c. Kiosk- A kiosk is a physical structure where products or services are sold or dispensed, such as connecting to a care provider using a computer touchscreen display.

d. Point-of-care devices - Point-of-care equipment is a type of medical equipment that can be used outdoors or in traditional healthcare environments, such as in medical camps or other activities.

e. Logistics- Transportation and distribution of medical goods and services, such as pharmaceuticals, medical supplies, medical devices and equipment, and other products, is referred to as logistics. Temperature readings, shock, moisture, and change of direction in pharmaceutical shipments are examples of IoMT applications; end-to-end visibility solutions that track personalized medicine for a specific cancer patient using radio-frequency identification (RFID) and barcodes; and drones that provide faster last-mile delivery are examples of IoMT applications.

In Clinic Segment

IoMT devices, which are utilised for administrative and clinical activities, are included in this segment. (At a clinic, through telehealth, or at the point of care). The InClinic segments of care devices differ from those in the community segment in a significant way.

Rather than the care provider physically using an instrument, here the trained staff uses the instrument. A variety of telehealth devices can be used to perform physical examinations, such as those of the heart, lungs, ears, skin, throat, and abdomen, and measurement of temperature.

Pros and Cons of IoMT

IoMT has a wide range of applications in the medical industry, ranging from patient devices to equipment and pharmaceutical supply chain management.

IoMT has demonstrated that it can transform the medical business from the groundup, though only time will tell whether that shift will be favorable or detrimental. This section discusses some of the pros and cons of IoMT [14].

Pros

Data in the Cloud & Predictive Analytics

Medications and medical equipment gather a massive amount of information every day, from vital signs to dosages to demographic data about the patients themselves. A vast amount of potential research data remains untouched, mainly since much of it is unsorted. Using predictive analytics, IoT devices enable the collection, sifting, and turning of information into valuable predictions. A single server receives all of the data, and predictive algorithms are applied to bring all this information together to conclude from seemingly unrelated data sets. Analyzing raw data can accurately predict diagnostic trends, drug usages, and even disease outbreaks. Diabetes patients should have their blood glucose levels checked, and a variety of IoT devices are already being used in hospitals around the country to improve patient care. When a patient tries to shift positions or leave their bed, smart beds record it. Health concerns can be tracked using smart tablets. RFID-enabled pill bottles that track when a patient takes their medication

Cons

Concerns About Patient Privacy and Security Breaches

The medical field now uses IoT technology to design the next generation of implantable medical devices, such as pacemakers and other devices. Newer pacemakers do not require a landline phone and bulky external device to be monitored; the device can be controlled simply by sending a Wi-Fi signal. In addition to keeping track of the implanted devices, doctors will receive alerts if the devices experience any malfunction. There are concerns about patient privacy raised by this. An insurance fraud case in Ohio led to police obtaining a search warrant for pacemaker data belonging to a suspect. Even though the search proved, the suspect committed fraud, using medical data as evidence sets a dangerous precedent.

BLOCKCHAIN TWINNING WITH AI AND IOT IN HEALTHCARE

Block chain is a popular study topic these days, and it can be used in a multitude of IoT scenarios. The Blockchain's significant qualities, such as decentralization, immutability, security and privacy, and transparency, are just a few of the primary reasons for its use in healthcare systems. Fig. (**5**) shows how AI and IoT fits in the workflow of Blockchain Technology in Healthcare Domain.

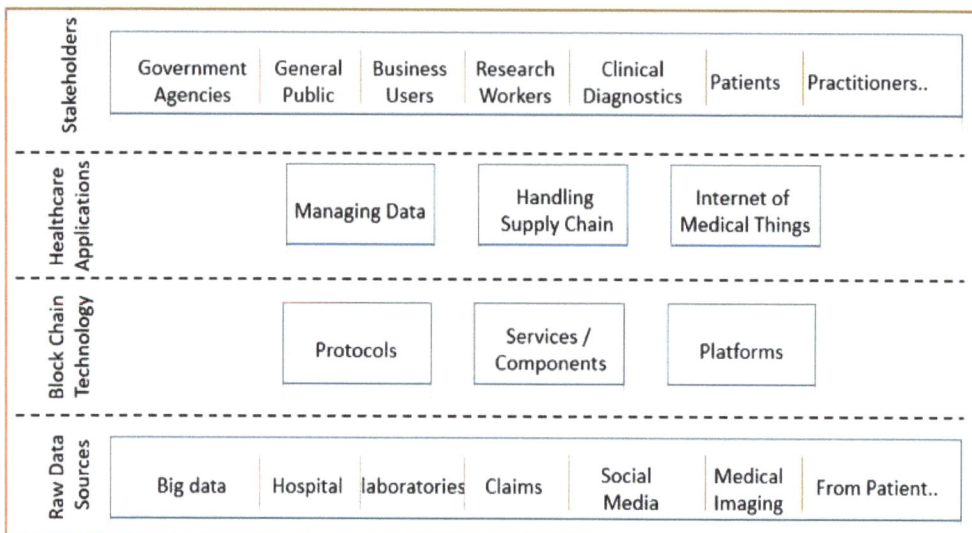

Fig. (5). The block chain workflow in healthcare.

There are mainly 4 layers in the Blockchain: Raw Data, Blockchain Technology, Healthcare Applications and Stakeholders.The IoT with AI provides flexibility in collecting information and doing predictive analysis.

As a decentralised technology, block chain allows multiple stakeholders to profit from healthcare applications. The Internet of Things, in particular one of its specialised domains, the Internet of Medical Things, is quickly becoming a major player in the healthcare domain.

Block chain and IoT are commonly used together to achieve decentralisation, privacy, and security in areas such as remote patient monitoring, electronic health records, and medical records management. `

CONCLUDING REMARKS

Due to the rise in medical care cost and the advancement in Artificial Intelligence and IoT, it is a welcome decision to adopt new tools and techniques and provide better treatment at the earliest. Thus, we hope to encounter constrained employment of AI in healthcare in the years to come. It is prominent that these AI tools are not going to replace physicians but rather are going to help them in decision-making and fastening the process.

Artificial intelligence (AI) and IoT have received enhanced attention in recent years, intending to solve complex problems. Similarly, the vast acceptance of artificial intelligence (AI) in healthcare is drastically transforming healthcare delivery. Artificial intelligence is applied in a range of settings, including hospitals, clinical laboratories, and healthcare staff. Machine-learning approaches using artificial intelligence have provided clinical practitioners and health service providers with previously unrealized opportunities. The chapter has presented the facets of AI and IoT in healthcare.

ACKNOWLEDGEMENTS

The chapter's inception, design, content, and flow of the chapter were all contributed by all authors. Each author contributed significantly to the chapter's preparation, reading, and final version.

REFERENCES

[1]   T. Lysaght, H.Y. Lim, V. Xafis, and K.Y. Ngiam, "AI-assisted decision-making in healthcare", *Asian Bioeth. Rev.,* vol. 11, no. 3, pp. 299-314, 2019.
        [http://dx.doi.org/10.1007/s41649-019-00096-0] [PMID: 33717318]

[2]   <https://data-flair.training/blogs/ai-in-healthcare-sector/> [Accessed 24 October 2021]

[3]   S. Kumar, P. Tiwari, and M. Zymbler, "Internet of Things is a revolutionary approach for future technology enhancement: a review", *Journal of Big Data,* vol. 6, no. 1, p. 111, 2019.
        [http://dx.doi.org/10.1186/s40537-019-0268-2]

[4]   A. Bohr, and K. Memarzadeh, *The rise of artificial intelligence in healthcare applications.* Artificial Intelligence in Healthcare Academic Press, 2020, pp. 25-60.
        [http://dx.doi.org/10.1016/B978-0-12-818438-7.00002-2]

[5]   S. Kumar, R.D. Raut, and B.E. Narkhede, "A proposed collaborative framework by using artificial intelligence-internet of things (AI-IoT) in COVID-19 pandemic situation for healthcare workers", *International Journal of Healthcare Management,* vol. 13, no. 4, pp. 337-345, 2020.
        [http://dx.doi.org/10.1080/20479700.2020.1810453]

[6]   "Ai and iot blended - what it is and why it matters?", Available at: https://www.clariontech.com/blog/ai-and-iot-blended-what-it-is-and-why-it-matters(Accessed on: 16 October 2021).

[7]   B. Wired, "Bringing the power of AI to the Internet of Things"", Available at: https://www.wired.com/brandlab/2018/05/bringing-power-ai-internet-things/(Accessed on: 16 August 2021).

[8]   G. Pardee, "Classifying patients to predict staff requirements", *The American Journal of Nursing,,* vol. 68, no. 3, pp. 517-520, 1968.
        [http://dx.doi.org/10.2307/3453442] [PMID: 5183559]

[9]   M. Dadkhah, M. Mehraeen, F. Rahimnia, and K. Kimiafar, "Use of internet of things for chronic disease management: An overview", *J. Med. Signals Sens.,* vol. 11, no. 2, pp. 138-157, 2021.
        [http://dx.doi.org/10.4103/jmss.JMSS_13_20] [PMID: 34268102]

[10]   I. Kayla Matthews, "How ai and iot are changing daily operations in hospitals", Available at: https://www.hcinnovationgroup.com/   analytics-ai/article/21132663/   how-ai-and-iot-are-cha-ging-daily-operations-in-hospitals(Accessed on: 16 August 2021).

[11] R. Stokke, "The personal emergency response system as a technology innovation in primary health care services: an integrative review", *J. Med. Internet Res.,* vol. 18, no. 7, p. e187, 2016.
[http://dx.doi.org/10.2196/jmir.5727] [PMID: 27417422]

[12] Jeremy Tucker, Available at: https://www.dronesinhealthcare.com/ Available at: https://www.drones-inhealthcare.com/(Accessed on: 16 September 2021).

[13] "The alliance of advanced biomedical engineering", Available at: https://aabme.asme.org/(Accessed: 23-May-2022).

[14] G.J. Joyia, R.M. Liaqat, A. Farooq, and S. Rehman, "Internet of medical things (iomt): applications, benefits and future challenges in healthcare domain", *J. of Comm.,* vol. 12, pp. 240-247, 2017.
[http://dx.doi.org/10.12720/jcm.12.4.240-247]

CHAPTER 5

Role of Social Media Platforms to Maintain Social Distancing in COVID-19 Pandemic

Sivakumar Vengusamy[1,*] and **Danapriya Visvanathan**[1]

[1] *School of Computing and Technology, Asia Pacific University of Technology and Innovation, Kuala Lumpur, Malaysia*

Abstract: Though it has been some time since the outbreak of the novel COVID-19 disease, it still poses a threat to many people worldwide. Connections have been lost due to the practice of social distancing, both on a personal and a societal level. Due to the global prohibitions on large-scale face-to-face meetings and activities, social media platforms have emerged as a lifesaver for humanity. The role of social media platforms has grown increasingly important for people to express themselves and communicate with others. Besides, the world has also witnessed large-scale events being organized on social media platforms, making connections and interactions with friends, family, and the community *via* social media networks, as well as the transformation of educational activities into digital activities. Thus, it is pertinent to comprehend the role of social media platforms in maintaining social distancing and online connections during the COVID-19 pandemic. This research aims to generate a discussion on the importance and role of social media platforms to maintain social distancing among individuals. It typically emphasizes three main themes: (1) the importance of social media platforms in establishing as well as improving social distancing during the COVID-19 crisis, (2) the role of social media platforms in maintaining social connections and interactions among individuals during the pandemic, and (3) the impact of Coronavirus towards the use of social media.

Keywords: Communication, Coronavirus, COVID-19, Disease, Facebook, Infection, Instagram, lockdown, Medical information, Pandemic, Physical distance, Role, Social distancing, Social isolation, Platforms, Social media, Virtual gathering, Virus, WhatsApp, YouTube.

INTRODUCTION

The Coronavirus disease 2019 (COVID-19) is a virus-related sickness that is now known as severe acute respiratory syndrome coronavirus 2 (SARS-CoV-2) [1]. COVID-19 is an infectious disease that causes mild to moderate respiratory

---

[*] **Corresponding Author Sivakumar Vengusamy:** School of Computing and Technology, Asia Pacific University of Technology and Innovation, Kuala Lumpur, Malaysia; Tel: ++91-9841253283, +91-9032874872; E-mail: dr.sivakumar@staffemail.apu.edu.my

sickness in most persons who are infected and recover without needing specific treatment. However, older people with medical issues such as cancer, chronic respiratory disease, diabetes, and cardiovascular disease are more prone to be infected with COVID-19 that can become a serious illness [2].

As a result, being well-informed about the virus is the safest method to avoid its transmission, the health issues it causes, and how to slow down its transmission. It is vital for people to protect themselves and others around them from being infected by washing hands, frequently using a hand sanitizer, wearing a face mask, and practicing social distancing. Social distancing is becoming an extremely important practice to be carried out in the course of slowing down the transmission of the virus mainly because when someone infected with the COVID-19 virus sneezes or coughs, the virus spreads predominantly through saliva droplets or nasal discharge.

Furthermore, experts from the health departments have analyzed the previous pandemics that have taken place and found that the spread of the virus is followed by the consequences of having large gatherings such as festivals and events, whereby people tend to spend more time physically close to each other. Thus, health experts believe that implementing interventions by banning people from being present in crowded places would significantly slow down the transmission of the disease [3], consequently, importance is given to social distancing.

The term social distancing also known as physical distancing is a public health practice that typically points out the measures to be taken for keeping a physical space between persons to avoid the spread of the contagious disease. The technique is primarily meant to prevent sick people from getting into close contact with healthy people. Besides, as COVID-19 can spread in a poorly ventilated environment in indoor settings, in which people usually spend a longer amount of time, physical distancing is vital to safeguard us from the virus.

Apart from that, another important reason to practice social distancing is mainly the lack of information and surety about who has been infected with the disease. One of the studies conducted based on the Wuhan statistics indicated that an estimated 59% of infected individuals were out and about, unknowingly infecting other individuals around them [4]. Many of the individuals who are infected with the virus did not show any symptoms. In that sense, there is a high possibility that 50% out of all COVID-19 cases could stay unnoticed as there are no insignificant symptoms. Therefore, people must practice social distancing by staying at home.

Staying at home can be practiced in various ways, such as closing schools, not allowing dining in at restaurants, having people to do work from home instead of being physically present at the workstation, and hosting a virtual party instead of having mass gatherings [5]. Besides, while these measures secure physical distance between individuals and reduce contact with contaminated surfaces, it eventually encourages virtual connections among individuals with families and communities in the outside world *via* the help of the platforms for social media.

SOCIAL MEDIA AS DISEASE CONTROL IN TIMES OF PANDEMIC

The majority of countries across the globe have been managing the COVID-19 pandemic *via* the implementation and practice of social distancing strategies. Subsequently, this led to an increase in the utilization of social media platforms, whereby many started depending on platforms such as Microsoft Teams and Zoom to stay connected for social, educational, and work purposes [6]. Social media typically describes the creation and exchange of information, ideas, and other kinds of expression through a virtual network or community using computer-mediated technology [7].

Examples of major social media networks are Instagram, Facebook, Twitter, LinkedIn, WhatsApp, WeChat, YouTube, Netflix, *etc.* With social media platforms playing a fundamental role in every individual's daily life, the way people communicate has been dramatically altered. It has become one of the most important tools for the government and public health organizations to provide people with accurate information mainly because social media has become increasingly important in spreading health information and policy announcements,.

A qualitative analysis has been carried out by Li *et al.* [8] to find out how government officials have utilized Twitter for anything related to the COVID-19 pandemic. The findings of the analysis revealed that out of 203 tweets, 48 tweets were more related to resources from the official government, while 166 tweets were informational, 19 tweets were related to boosting self-confidence, and 14 tweets were more politically related. Furthermore, another study carried out by Merkley *et al.* [9] shows that the term 'Coronavirus' has become the recent trend from the searched terms.

This is where importance was given more related to the measures to be taken in practicing proper hygiene as well as maintaining physical distancing to cope with the COVID-19 pandemic.

Apart from that, Wang *et al.* [10] also found that some studies investigated in their research show that a huge number of YouTube videos were created about the COVID-19 disease prevention methods, whereby it is categorized into four different groups such as washing hands, face mask-wearing, social distancing, and risk assessments.

Another cross-sectional research carried out by Basch *et al.* [11] presents that there were about 100 videos on the YouTube channel which are listed as the top videos with the greatest number of views that have been created and uploaded on the platform of January 2020 with the keyword 'Coronavirus'. These videos have had a total of 125 million views, whereby it also discloses that the average number of daily visits to YouTube has increased since January 2020. Social media has become a reliable platform to control the disease by distributing more information about coronavirus since the beginning of the COVID-19 pandemic and allowing individuals to stay connected.

TOP 3 REASONS FOR USING SOCIAL MEDIA PLATFORMS DURING THE PANDEMIC

The platforms for social media have become prevalently used by many individuals for various reasons during the times of a pandemic. However, the utilization of social media channels has rapidly increased since the government has ordered the public to stay at home as much as possible to avoid face to face interactions to break the chain of infections. Fig. (**1**) on the following page shows the percentage of users who has been spending a longer hour on social media platforms for various activities due to the COVID-19 pandemic.

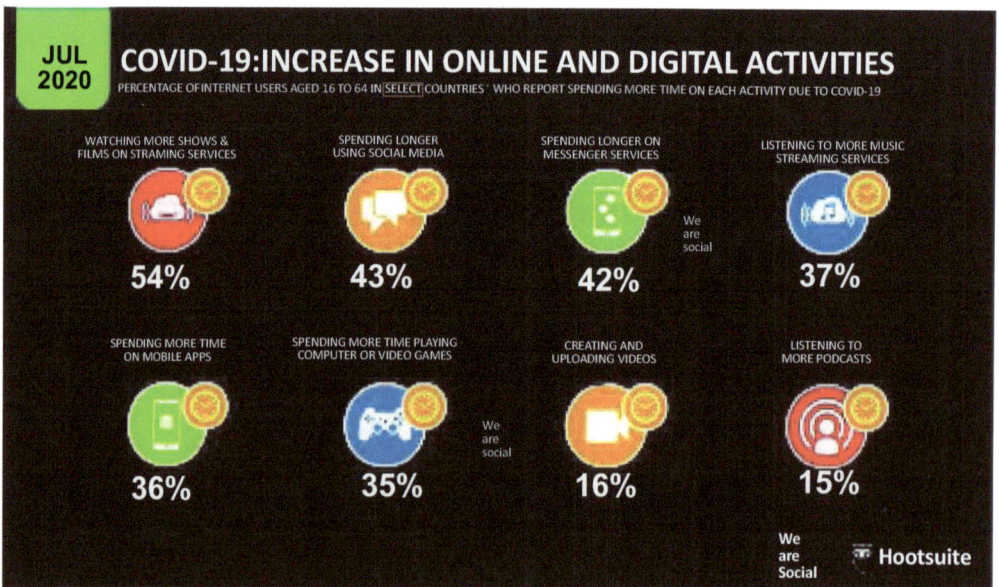

Fig. (1). The Percentage of Users Spending Longer Time on Social Media Platforms for Various Activities [12].

The top reasons for using social media channels by many include seeking information about the COVID-19 disease, self-entertainment due to the lockdown, and online shopping. These aspects are further discussed below.

Seeking for Information

The usage of social media platforms to look for information regarding the coronavirus disease, its related medical information, as well as the impacts of the virus not only involve people who are living in urban areas, but also individuals who live in remote areas, as the government of the respective countries around the world has made internet connection accessible to everyone. Besides, social media platforms have provided a huge number of chances to people all over the world to participate in and contribute to online communities. This can be useful for every individual by gaining and collecting more information about the COVID-19 outbreak situation both locally and at the global level.

Furthermore, social media platforms have connected most individuals across the globe *via* Instagram, Facebook, Twitter, WhatsApp, Line, and YouTube. These online platforms are extremely useful for people to get their daily updates especially regarding the COVID-19 pandemic [13]. Besides, Fig. (**2**) below shows that studies have revealed that most people are considering using WhatsApp to obtain accurate information especially during the pandemic, compared to other online platforms for social media. Instagram, Facebook, Line, and YouTube are useful for people in order to share information as well as to be aware of the pandemic.

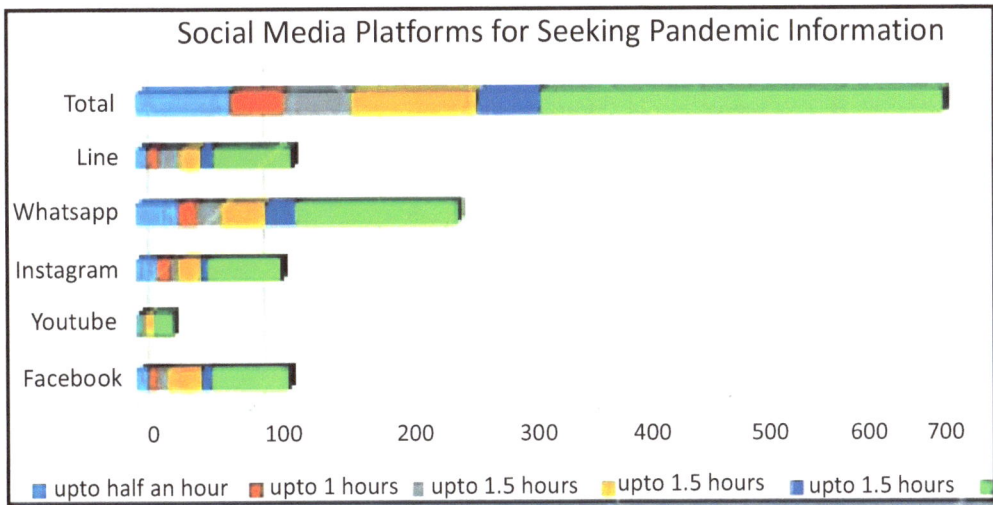

Fig. (2). Social Media Platforms Used for Seeking Pandemic Information [14].

Most people have indicated that they have been utilizing online social media platforms regularly to check for current updates regarding the COVID-19 pandemic. Consequently, this clearly shows that the utilization of social media benefits many individuals by providing news updates and a learning platform about the COVID-19 disease. In support of this, an analysis was carried out by Saud M. *et al* [14], showing that the vast majority of those who took part in the survey agreed that social media platforms have benefitted people to various extents including being a useful source of learning and gathering information about the disease [15].

In addition, most people across the globe are conscious of the fact that social media sites are indeed helping them to be updated with the latest information about the coronavirus disease as well as that social media has changed their behavior regarding taking precautionary steps towards their safety as well as their family's safety.

Entertainment

Additionally, social media platforms are also widely used by most people for entertainment reasons to reduce stress and to facilitate staying at home during the pandemic days. An analysis carried out by Trifonova V [16]. shows that young people are the most active users of social media sites to keep themselves occupied during the pandemic. Besides, TikTok is one of the well-known platforms for social media that is serving people with tons of entertaining and funny videos that attract individuals to use the platform to fill up their spare time.

The idea of using social media platforms to fill up my spare time has excited me for quite some time. Since the COVID-19 epidemic began, the focus of using social media channels to absorb content passively has now extended its focus to individuals also creating content. TikTok, as mentioned earlier, being one of the most popular platforms for video content, is the platform that has been used extensively by people to create and upload videos compared to other platforms such as Facebook, Instagram, or Twitter. Online activities, such as creating and uploading videos on TikTok that have been accelerated recently by the pandemic, have become the reason for increasing social media engagement since April 2020.

Research shows that TikTok is one of the social networking sites with a huge spike of visitors in which the application acts as the main facilitator for viral video sharing by people around the world. Apart from that, social media platforms have also attracted various people looking for ways to adapt to their circumstances such as taking care of kids while having to perform other responsibilities and experiencing a higher level of work stress due to the lockdown. This is where new parents with babies as well as parents with younger children, are found to be generating and uploading videos more on the social media platforms that are declared as video-sharing sites mainly due to the pandemic.

Shopping

Another top reason for the growing utilization of social media platforms during the COVID-19 outbreak is online shopping. Most people these days are using various social media channels for shopping [17]. Social media platforms have not only grown to facilitate sharing of the latest news and updates about the pandemic, as well as entertainment, however, shopping has also become one of the highest online behaviors. This does not imply that people are opting to shop online primarily due to the COVID-19 outbreak; millions of people are found to purchase products online even before the occurrence of the pandemic. Thus, social media platforms are been to be a fundamental part of a huge number of online shopping customer's habits for quite some time.

Moreover, social media platforms have become a common channel that aids individuals daily to obtain information about products of any brand. In fact, since more of the products nowadays are being advertised online for purchasing since the lockdown, a huge number of e-commerce users have purchased products newly based on their discoveries made over social media platforms [18]. Furthermore, products discovered online by consumers are immensely based on the brand's presence on such platforms.

Social media channels typically hold an essential role in consumer's decision-making process to consider a specific brand. In addition, social media appearance also impacts consumers' decisions to purchase products from a particular brand. This is where online sellers are responsible for ensuring that their product pages look and feel good for their potential customers. This is mainly due to the reason that many consumers visit the brand's profile on social media channels before deciding to purchase its products. Consequently, this clearly shows that social media platforms have turned to help people by keeping them entertained and engaged while maintaining social distancing to slow down the spread of the coronavirus disease.

DISCUSSION

Importance of Social Media Platforms in Establishing As Well As Improving Social Distancing During the COVID-19 Crisis

The disastrous situation caused by the COVID-19 pandemic has made most countries to impose schooling and working from home periods that started in March 2020. Though many countries have lifted these conditional movement orders by January 2021 [19], several countries have been still extending the orders till now June 2021 due to the third wave of the disease. However, people's activities over the Internet have increased mainly to fund their activities at home during the pandemic *via* the usage of smartphones. Besides, it is also interesting to point out that this is the first time a pandemic has been predominantly publicized *via* the Internet and social media platforms [20].

Spread of Information

One of the main importance of utilizing social media in times of pandemic is to educate people around the world about the level of information being disseminated on online platforms compared to the information being provided *via* traditional methods such as newspaper articles. The use of social media channels to educate people about the Coronavirus disease also has great significance due to the rapid circulation of information.

Besides, a number of data analysts across the globe who have developed infographics that relate to confirmed and suspected COVID-19 patients have shared their data over social media platforms such as WeChat and Twitter [21]. In a few days since the infographics were shared, a huge number of requests have been received to translate the content into more than ten different languages [21], which clearly shows the speed of information traveling around the world through social media.

Furthermore, the World Health Organization (WHO), a very well-trusted health organization, uses social media platforms to post substantiated information to inform the public about the disease. It is shocking to know that information is shared across social media channels such as Twitter, Facebook, and Instagram by leaders to ensure correct information and knowledge about the disease is being circulated around to people. Moreover, the government has also been interacting with people actively over social media to ensure no false information is disseminated during the pandemic.

Besides that, WhatsApp, which has been utilized commonly for social communication these days, has gained a powerful stand for sharing information. More and more people are creating several dedicated group chats over the instant messaging application, in which information is being shared instantly and extensively. Many individuals who have joined these groups were getting of at least 200 messages on WhatsApp in the early stages of the COVID-19 epidemic. The type of WhatsApp messages that have been circulating includes protocols as well as updates that relate to the well-being of people. Likewise, Fig. (**3**) below shows several sample messages shared on social media platforms.

Guidelines/Protocols/SOPs

- A ward round checklist for intensive care was created in Cardiff and refined by sharing on social media, incorporating helpful suggestions.
- A checklist on using anaesthetic machines as ICU ventilators was created in Birmingham and widely distributed on social media platforms.
- Some advice and an informal algorithm by two Italian intensivists from the Lombardy region involved in the surge since the first local outbreak have been designed into an infographic with the purpose of supporting physicians caring for patients with severe COVID-19 induced respiratory failure, so as to standardise their approach, thereby optimising outcome and resources consumption. Based solely on the original post on Twitter, the Italian version of the infographic has to-date generated 11,836 impressions and 761 reactions, with the English translation generating 49,548 impressions, with 5508 engagements.
- An infographic on the principles of airway management in COVID-19 incorporating infection control procedures to reduce the transmission risk of SARS-CoV-2 infection was drafted by the Anaesthesia and Intensive Care Department of the Prince of Wales Hospital in Hong Kong. This was translated into 17 languages through collaborations with colleagues and centres internationally.
- A single email written after a COVID-19 briefing was shared on Whatsapp, disseminated through multiple Whatsapp groups and eventually appeared on social media platforms where it was shared by thousands of users, much to the bemusement of the intensivist who wrote the email.

Fig. (3). Sample Messages Shared on Social Media Platform [7].

Creating Awareness

Apart from that, creating awareness about COVID-19 among individuals is also an important role of social media platforms during the pandemic to educate people while maintaining social distancing. With the measures taken by the government to advise people to confine themselves to their homes during the pandemic, a huge number of individuals have taken the initiative to play a part over social media channels to create awareness about the COVID-19 pandemic.

Among them includes well-known celebrities who have been utilizing their standing to help raise awareness among the public. This is where a challenge comes known as the Safe Hands Challenge program that has been spreading over social media platforms as one of the efforts taken by the influencers to educate their audience on the value and necessity of personal hygiene. Besides, to raise awareness of the COVID-19 disease, WHO has partnered with TikTok, a popular video-sharing app.

Accurate Understanding

Besides, social media channels also allow organizations to obtain an accurate understanding of their customer's requirements during the COVID-19 pandemic. Since the government has encouraged most people to stay at home to stop the spread of COVID-19 illness, most organizations have moved to online platforms to continue doing their business. In this effort, social media platforms have been playing the biggest part for organizations to identify their potential customer's views and opinions and to coordinate with them. This is where through the utilization of social media, companies can easily engage with their customers *via* social media private chats, groups, as well as comment sections.

With social media platforms, organizations can also gather a wide range of information such as customer information and latest events. This information will then be able to be used by companies to track and examine customers' views regarding the particular business or products on social media. Customer's views in this regard would include complaints, feedback, and suggestions. These views would consequently serve as a guide for organizations to further improve their businesses and carry out the necessary alterations that would result in greater customer satisfaction. Likewise, companies are also able to interact with their customers by requesting input as well as providing prompt responses to inquiries or complaints *via* the usage of social media platforms.

Business Costs Saving

Social media platforms also enable businesses to save costs during the pandemic. This is where typical market research by organizations takes a long time and costs a lot of money. However, since businesses have now moved to the online platforms, the social media has been utilized as an extensive tool by organizations to acquire insights into their dedicated market, branding, customers, and other essential factors in the market research. Market research over social media platforms consequently improves the efficacy of the company's marketing strategies as the speed of obtaining knowledge about their target market through social media is rapid compared to the traditional method.

Besides, the social media platforms that have been used widely by organizations include Twitter, Instagram, and Facebook in order to conduct market research and track down the trends in the market. Subsequently, organizations can obtain insights into the emerging trends by just having a look through people's most recent posts and the popular terms used by their potential customers and distinguish customer opinions about their products and services in a real-time manner. Moreover, social media platforms also assist businesses in participating in open discussions with their potential customers. This research technique eventually enables organizations to collect important data and gain an intense understanding of customers' views and preferences.

Additionally, the market research that organizations have carried out reveals that customers prefer advertisements over social media platforms compared to the traditional advertisements. Thus, using social media platforms for market research enables costs and energy saving which eventually reduces business costs compared to investing time and money in developing a marketing plan that does not have a clear outcome.

Role of Social Media Platforms in Maintaining Social Distancing during the Pandemic

Since the arrival of the coronavirus disease, millions of people have been making use of the available social media platforms more than what it was usual mainly due to the reason of seeking information about the disease as well as coping with the lockdown circumstances such as staying at home most of the time while carrying on their daily activities. These ultimately contribute to the effort of maintaining social distancing to disrupt the infectious chain. Besides, the use of social media platforms brings a great deal of relief to many people throughout the COVID-19 pandemic. Subsequently, this section discusses the social media platforms' roles in the context of maintaining social distancing among people during the outbreak.

A Source of Medical Information

One of the roles of social media platforms in maintaining social distancing includes being a source to gather medical information about the coronavirus. The COVID-19 disease has been developing quickly, in which guidelines and strategies created by the governments, as well as health organizations, are continuously progressing in consideration of the evidence that has been gathered up to date [22]. This justifies the need for information to be shared quickly and efficiently. In that sense, social media platforms have grown into an increasingly well-known source of information in medical.

The rapid dissemination of resources over social media channels is one of the significant characteristics of the platform. This is where in a study conducted by Chan *et al* [23], the authors mentioned that an infographic related to protecting healthcare professionals against the coronavirus disease was posted on platforms such as WeChat and Twitter as well as on the hospital's official website. Consequently, their outcomes have pointed out that the speed of visiting and disseminating this sort of learning resources over social media platforms particularly on Twitter was much faster compared to websites [23]. Hence, due to the rapid knowledge-sharing feature, social media platforms are more effective and valuable in delivering information on time to people across the globe.

Moreover, social media has become a channel for everyone to obtain access to medical information, which ranges from information provided by healthcare professionals to information obtained from an amateur person's experiences towards well-being and disease. The social media platforms that are being utilized to disseminate information regarding the COVID-19 disease include YouTube, Twitter, internet forums, Facebook, and Instagram. This is where official government channels on Facebook, Instagram, and Twitter frequently publish the latest statistics on the number of recent infections together with advice that encourages people to adhere to the guidelines set to reduce the growing number of positive COVID-19 cases.

The popular terms "Stay Safe" and "Stay at Home" orders became famous *via* social media platforms [24], which indirectly supports the efforts to maintain social distancing. Furthermore, healthcare professionals have also made an effort to advertise medical information on social media sites that the majority of teenager's visit, such as TikTok, to enable the rapid sharing of information among people of all ages. Good personal hygiene is one of the most important habits that must be practiced by people to avoid contracting the COVID-19 illness. In order to guide people with good hygiene practices, many videos are created and uploaded over the YouTube channel that demonstrates the right-hand methods to the public.

YouTube is also being used to educate health professionals to follow proper techniques to put on their personal protective gear. There are also forums that allow doctors to share their knowledge about diseases based on evidence while providing support to their coworkers. Besides, the social media network plays a significant role in making valid information universally available for people across the globe. The characteristic of online social media platforms allows medical information to be easily updated and shared, whereby is essential at the beginning stage of the coronavirus outbreak. Also, regardless of the challenges brought over by social media, such as invalidated information, the platforms still play a great role in maintaining and managing social distancing in times of the pandemic.

Social Media for Online Education

Subsequently, another role of social media platforms in maintaining social distancing includes facilitating online education. Social media platforms have enabled communication during which the students, and educational institution members, were isolated in support of maintaining social distancing to share important information [25]. Since the existence of the coronavirus disease in 2020, educational institutions have experienced an enormous shift from traditional classrooms to online platforms, where one can learn from the convenience of one's own home. While the role of social media channels towards education is not a new thing, it seems to have been moved from concept by the majority to action since last year as the pandemic has compelled people to try out new ways of learning to maintain social distancing, consequently staying safe from the disease.

The new normal introduced by the government involves an attempt to make the most of the implementation of online education. Furthermore, it ultimately benefits students from non-green zones the most, as it aids in breaking the chain of infection in severely impacted areas by preserving social distance. Moreover, when it comes to online education, the platform for social media allows for sharing resources for learning purposes, consequently leading to modern learning. Apart from maintaining social distancing, studies indicate that incorporating social media platforms with teaching and learning environment would eventually allow new patterns of communication, collaboration and social impacts among students and tutors [26].

A study conducted by Balakrishnan & Gan [27]. discusses that the admiration towards social media motivates learning mainly due to its immense recognition and its capability to allow virtual education groups that eventually encourage vigorous interaction between tutors and students. There are also several studies which have been carried out on the application of social media platforms for various reasons in the education system, such as supporting student engagement and the process of learning, developing a network, as well as intellectual communication [28].

The outcomes of the studies exhibited that the platforms for social media, such as WhatsApp and Facebook, were the utmost tools used to carry out formal communication between students and university department members. The good perception that social media platforms have created among students allows them to perceive the online channels as an easy-to-use, interactive and worthwhile tools. It clearly shows that the utilization of social media platforms for online education eventually supports social distancing, social existence and learning.

Since the education ministries in respective countries have ordered all the educational institutions to conduct online classes due to the confinement imposed by the COVID-19 pandemic, schools and universities have also begun to incorporate social media platforms such as Google Classroom, Facebook Live as well as Zoom to facilitate online classes. Separate groups for students from a given semester were created for both the Facebook Live and Google Meet sessions. In addition, the Facebook Live sessions seemed to be a more convenient and user-friendly way of learning for students and tutors as it does not necessarily need any pre-requisite skills [29]. Fig. (**4**) below typically illustrates a basic online education model for students during the COVID-19 pandemic.

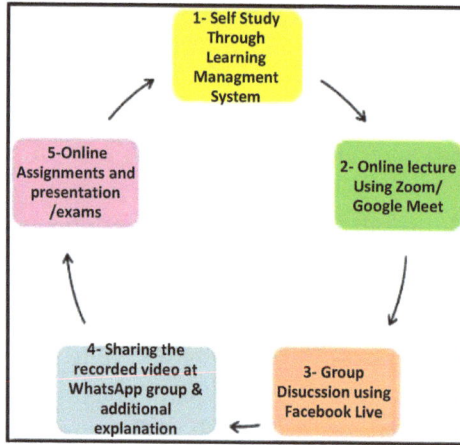

Fig. (4). Online Education Model for Students during the Pandemic [29].

YouTube as a Learning Platform

Many individuals have also utilized youtube as a learning resource these days. The online video platform has transformed itself to become completely customizable and provide an interactive video experience for users. Hence, YouTube consequently motivates user creativity. Moreover, one of the main features of YouTube is to allow users to share videos with people. This characteristic of the platform directly benefits the students, whereby the channel can play a role in sharing educational content among the students while maintaining social distancing. This is where YouTube typically allows access to various educational videos without requiring any fee.

Additionally, YouTube can build an enjoyable learning environment among students. It not only allows students to connect with their schoolmates and respective educators *via* the network, but it also allows them to connect with students and tutors across the globe [30]. Also, students will be able to view, download, and share educational videos such as instructional videos, science and exploration, scientific discoveries, *etc.* with other students. YouTube is one of the social media platforms due to the reason that it allows sharing of video content which subsequently allows individuals to post their comments, which it indirectly stimulate communication to take place. It makes learning more effective for students. It is also because YouTube eventually allows students to communicate and collaborate with each other on the platform to develop their problem-solving and decision-making skills [31]. In support of these, a number of studies revealed that YouTube channels have well assisted online education. A study performed by Iqbal *et al.* [32] shows that YouTube was a platform used by students as a substitute to carry out online learning.

Besides, an exploration conducted by Dewi & Carniasih [33]. also revealed that videos uploaded and shared *via* YouTube have assisted students in maintaining social distancing by staying at home in a way that the platform can allow videos to reach a huge number of people in one single presentation at different locations simultaneously.

Instagram as a Learning Platform

Instagram is another social media network that many people uses as a learning resource. Based on the usage level of Instagram by online users, it indicates that the platform's popularity level has not decreased as well and will not show any sign of annihilation anytime soon when compared with other social media platforms. Besides, Instagram is a social networking platform that allows users to upload and share photographs and videos with other Instagram users. This particular feature of the platform has consequently attracted hundreds of millions of people worldwide to use social media for various reasons.

Educators can also perceive this opportunity as an online learning resource to support social isolation during the COVID-19 pandemic. Instagram is an application that can be downloaded and installed on mobile devices to facilitate a potent learning experience. Principally to support learning experiences that are carried out based on technologies, individuals are recommended to make use of the available technologies such as tablets, iPads, smartphones, as well as other appropriate mobile devices that can have positive effects on the process of online teaching and learning.

Instagram is well known to be one of the social media channels that encourage technology-based learning [34] while also maintaining social distancing. A study carried out by Shazali *et al.* [35] revealed that Instagram has aided students in developing their writing skills in the context of a rise in the level of interest to learn and new vocabulary. As the phrase goes 'A picture is worth a thousand words'; with simple media such as Instagram, students will be more interested to learn things. In addition, an experiment performed by Supiandi *et al* [36] shows that individuals can improve their high-order thinking skills with the use of Instagram by an average of 94%.

In support of the experiment by Supiandi Manaroinsong [37]. has also found that Instagram has the potential to improve higher-order thinking abilities in individuals and to develop individual creativity and social skills while learning about technologies. As a result, these studies, show that Instagram can be used for the process of blended learning as well as online education while staying at home.

WhatsApp as a Learning Platform

The majority of people have also used WhatsApp as a medium for learning. It is an application that facilitates cross-platform instant messaging on mobile devices. WhatsApp allows text, audio, video, and images to be shared instantly in a real-time to a particular individual and a group of people without requiring any fee. Besides, integrating WhatsApp in the field of education typically offers students as well as teachers an interface that can be used easily. This is where students will be able to receive notifications instantly about course updates and learning materials *via* WhatsApp. WhatsApp also provides a news feed and allows users to respond on time.

Apart from that, learning *via* WhatsApp is recommended to be applied at various levels of education in order to encourage social distancing among the learning community in regard to the pandemic [38]. Other than breaking the chain of infection, it consequently allows students to learn from anywhere at any time using their mobile devices. In support of this statement, a study conducted by Alenazi [39]. mentions that the WhatsApp application can also be utilized also as a tool to share academic information *via* group or private chats in the form of voice messages, images, videos, as well as documents. Moreover, the platform also can distribute recorded lecture sessions to students over group chats to assist them with revisions.

A study indicates that by using this approach, students were also able to improve their communication skills by working with their tutors more effectively than classroom learning. The instant messaging application enables three different types of interactions to be taken place among the learning community such as students interacting with the course content, students interacting with peers, as well as tutors interacting among them. The implementation of WhatsApp in education essentially serves as a valuable platform to facilitate learning, teaching and communication that subsequently aids in maintaining social distancing during the pandemic.

A Marketing Platform

Apart from aiding education, social media also plays an important and effective role in the marketing industry to maintain social distancing in times of the COVID-19 pandemic. Organizations in the marketing field often utilize platforms for social media that can offer a different kind of advertising features to promote their products and services. Though digital marketing is not a new term these days, the usage of social media platforms for marketing communication to be taken place has increased during the pandemic to maintain social distancing.

Social media marketing characteristically does not require a huge number of financial resources when compared with the traditional approach, which requires the use of billboards and televisions. Organizations that practice social media marketing essentially require only mobile devices with an active internet connection [40] which eventually reduces costs in the long term. Furthermore, given the current situation, in which most people are compelled to stay at home, businesses must adapt their services by establishing new marketing techniques to enable their online social media clients to engage with their products from the comfort of their homes. Subsequently, this allows businesses and their customers to maintain social distancing while still interacting by purchasing products over social media channels along with available contact-free home delivery services. This approach also allows individuals to be able to get what they want as well as businesses to continue operating successfully.

Utilizing paid social media marketing is highly effective in promoting new products and services to both current and potential online customers especially during the pandemic. Using platforms such as Instagram and Facebook for advertising campaigns ultimately allows brands and products to reach targeted customers from a particular geographical area, age group, and people with a specific brand interest. Hence, marketing *via* social media platforms is considered the most cost -effective approach for organizations to successfully achieve their business goals. In addition, the outcome of social media marketing shows that brand recognition has increased significantly in times of the pandemic as it allows businesses to frequently interact with their customers, eventually enhancing their credibility.

Marketing on social media channels not only helps businesses to reach their local customers; nevertheless, it also allows them to get people from all around the world. Hence, keeping in mind today's situation, digital marketing over social media platforms is fundamentally the backbone of every organization to support the company's operational processes and procedures [41] until the pandemic ends. Generally speaking, utilizing social media platforms for marketing by organizations is an effective method to reduce operational costs while also keeping up with social distancing throughout the COVID-19 pandemic.

Positive Thinking

Another role of social media platforms in supporting social distancing during the COVID-19 pandemic is also helping people have positive thinking. This is mainly because social media platforms were able to share a lot of life-saving information, allow individuals to be connected over the network while staying at home, and create a sense of global unity. Moreover, social media platforms allow every individual to share their personal experiences with friends and family to assist them in fighting their emotions caused by being quarantined at home to maintain social distancing among the people. The social media channels also remind people that they are not alone instead, they can still stay connected with people over the network while breaking the chain of coronavirus infections.

One of the ways that social media platforms allow people to stay positive during the pandemic is by organizing and distributing fundraisers over the network to assist people in need to raise money [42]. The coronavirus pandemic has put a huge number of people in challenging situations such as working parents who have to take care of their kids while working from home as daycare centers have been ordered to be closed, disabled people, as well as people who have lost their jobs. Also, in times of the COVID-19 pandemic, a group of people stayed united to support individuals and organizations by distributing fundraisers among their large circle of friends over social media channels.

In addition, social media platforms have also been utilized by people to offer support to people in need, such as helping those who are unable to leave their homes to pick up groceries as well as share information with people who are struggling to run their local businesses. Likewise, as mentioned earlier, posting images and videos of their experiences over social media platforms has also enabled people to develop a positive mindset to cope with the situation and stay at home during the lockdown. The pictures and videos posted over social media ranged from pictures and videos of their pets who were excited to have their owners staying and playing with them all day to videos of people doing yoga postures.

Impact of Coronavirus on the Use of Social Media

In addition, despite the roles that social media platforms play during the pandemic, as discussed in the earlier section, there is still a lot more to learn about the impact that the coronavirus can bring on the use of social media platforms by individuals. It is very well known that this is the first time any generation has ever experienced a widespread virus of this scale. The below section discusses several impacts that the pandemic has brought on using social media platforms to maintain social distancing.

The Social Media Participation

Through a number of analyses carried out by researchers, it is found that more and more people have started using social media channels and spending more of their time staying online while using social media platforms on a routine basis. This is mainly due to the consequences that the pandemic has brought. Thus, to cope with the situation, people began to occupy their time by using the internet more and more, which has eventually increased social media utilization.

Moreover, according to several reports, almost 50% of adults in America have begun to use social media platforms, with the average amount of duration spent online over social media channels has increased by an hour every day than usually, it is in times of the pandemic [43]. Up to the present moment, reports indicated that Facebook had been the most prominent social media platform being used by online users, which is then followed by.

Instagram, as well as TikTok. Besides, since the amount of time spent on social media platforms has been increasing recently caused by he physical restrictions and the social distancing policy, many individuals are also participating in online advertisements.

One of the investigations found that the number of online users who participate in online advertisements has increased by 15%, especially during the pandemic [43]. In addition, according to another estimate, the influence of social media platforms has increased by 20%, indirectly indicating that the number of people using social media who are paying more attention to internet advertisements has risen. The report also mentions that this is a consequence due to online advertisements being posted on social media platforms in the form of videos and in the platform's story such as Facebook or Instagram story.

As more individuals are staying online most of the time in a day, business organizations have also started to make use of this opportunity to connect with their future customers. This is where organizations began to create entry through paid social advertisements over social media platforms to promote their products on sale. The pandemic has also allowed social media users to appreciate the increase in interactions between the users and the brands which has consequently allowed businesses to gain new customers [44].

Since the pandemic has resulted in following the social distancing policy imposed by the government, more users of social media platforms are instinctively motivated to look for social connections. Hence, many people are turning to the influencers oversocial media platforms, which has consequently increased their content due to the pandemic. Besides, according to one of the surveys that have been carried out, it is learned that more than 80% of social media users in the UK and the US have been observing more content in times of the pandemic.

The Social Media Demeanor

The coronavirus disease also has a great impact on the behaviors of online users. Since people are restricted from having physical interactions to contain the spread of the COVID-19 virus, the urge for live content that includes pictures and videos has increased. In support of this, social media platforms are attracting the online users with clips that are in the standard format and with a new format like IGTV and Facebook Watch. Fig. (**5**) below shows data collected recently from online users regarding their activities over social media platforms during the pandemic.

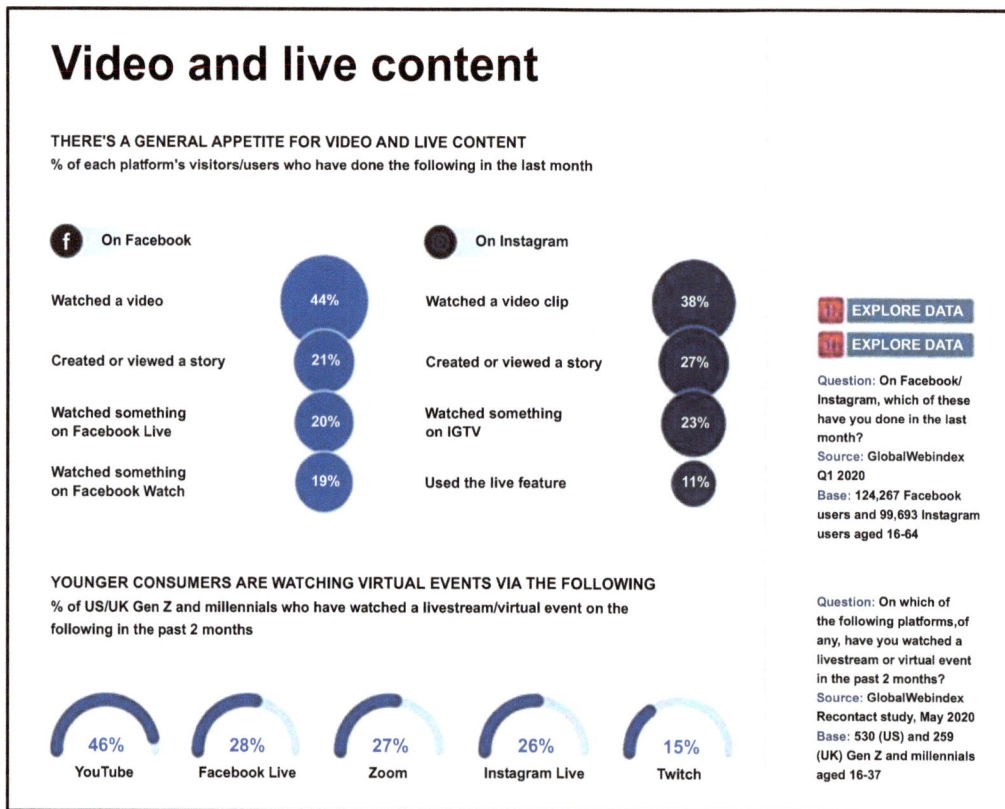

Fig. (5). Types of Behavior of the Social Media Users during the COVID-19 Pandemic [44].

Due to the restrictions enforced by the governments, there are a large group of people who have planned for celebrations such as weddings or birthday events to be conducted, which will not be allowed to be carried out with a huge group of people gathered at a specific location mainly due to COVID-19 disease. Hence, though the coronavirus disease impacts people negatively in this term, it had a positive impact *via* social media, whereby people have begun to use social media platforms for virtual gatherings. This is where many individuals can be invited to join a virtual event hosted online. Fig. (**5**) in the previous page also reveals that younger users are delighted to attend virtual events over various social media platforms.

Moreover, the social distancing rules imposed due to the pandemic have further motivated people to utilize social media tools like WhatsApp, Skype, or Zoom to have a catch up session with family members and friends. Most social media applications these days are now providing video conferencing features with anyone over the internet. Online users can hold a group video chat with more than two people who will be allowed to join the group call using most social media applications. Consequently, this aids people living in stress due to the circumstances of having to stay at home.For instance, having an evening tea time with a close friend over a Zoom video call. Hence, using social media applications for these purposes is becoming an instant mood enhancer during social isolation. This is especially true when users of social media platforms post stories on Facebook and Instagram that show pictures of having a video call session with friends and family members. Fig. (**6**) on the next page shows a screenshot of an individual sharing a story on his Instagram account about having a video call gathering with his friends in times of isolation.

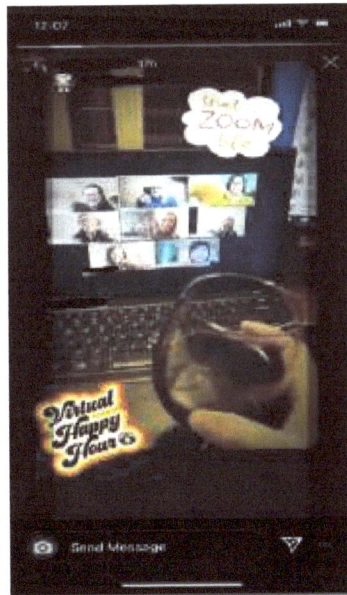

Fig. (6). An Example Screenshot of an Individual having a Virtual Gathering during Isolation [45].

In addition, since individuals are restricted to going out with family and friends for movie nights due to the social distancing rules, people have also started to utilize social media platforms to create a party environment *via* Netflix [45]. This is where individuals can create a movie night virtually over the Netflix application with their friends and family members even while being physically isolated to allow themselves to enjoy watching a movie with their loved ones.

The Online Shopping Journey

Though online shopping is not a new activity among internet users, it has been utilized more than the average usage of e-commerce websites. More and more people have started to shop online due to the widespread COVID-19 disease, due to which restrictions have been imposed for physical presence at stores. It typically aids individuals in purchasing items online with convenience and safety while staying at their homes, and avoiding crowded areas. Besides, online shopping has also been playing its role in allowing people to get what they want, which consequently helps to maintain social distancing among individuals.

Subsequently, buying and shopping online has made organizations expand their e-commerce business with new products and customers. A report shows that online sales have increased by 15.1%, and customers have spent about $10.8 billion during the pandemic. The report also indicated that these records have in fact broken the previous online purchasing records. Furthermore, as mentioned in the earlier section, social media platforms also enabled businesses to increase their brand discovery among consumers *via* online advertisements on social media mainly because the pandemic has caused people to spend more time on screens while staying at home.

The online advertisements posted by businesses over social media channels have also allowed people to have direct responses to their queries about the products that are put on sale. This has eventually made an impact on the younger generations whereby social media has become the go-to platform in search of their intended brands or products to be purchased. Moreover, the platforms for social media such as Instagram and Facebook highly encourage online users to consider it a place for shopping, whereby the platform contains a tab for shopping. It is discovered that 20% of Facebook users who are from all generations as well as demographics make use of the marketplace on Facebook on a monthly basis, which includes purchasing items such as clothes, gaming accessories, and furniture .

As a result, many small businesses have had the opportunity to reach their potential customers across the world *via* social media platforms. The pandemic of COVID-19 has the potential to bring an intense negative impact on businesses of all sizes if they remain running their businesses using the traditional approach. Hence, more and more commerce businesses have now started moving toward online platforms in running their business to embrace the new social distancing solutions such as shopping through WhatsApp.

CONCLUDING REMARKS

Simple social and communication rules to maintain social distance between persons might help to reduce coronavirus infection while also easing the demands placed on people due to the global economic situation. Thus, the government as well as the policymakers, have imposed policies about social networks. Social media platforms are an extremely valuable tool to be utilized for interaction between people in times of the pandemic and it allows interactions to take place between the government and the public. Besides, social media content can support the development and maintenance of the social distancing policy among individuals. This is where social media channels allow people access to information related to each individual's roles and responsibilities during the pandemic. Moreover, to maintain social distancing, social media platforms also play a role in offering ways to increase awareness of the COVID-19 disease as well as improve individual connections caused by physical isolation. Nevertheless, over-usage of social media platforms has also sparked considerable worry and anxiety about the COVID-19 pandemic, potentially harming humans' mental health and psychological well-being. Overall, the utilization of social media platforms has allowed social distancing policy to be implemented more successfully among the people. There are a huge number of benefits in using social media channels to communicate and distribute health related information during the pandemic, as well as maintaining social distancing that has enabled people to look for alternative ways to continue learning as well as working from home to break the chain of the coronavirus infection.

ACKNOWLEDGEMENTS

All authors contributed to the study conception and design. Material preparation, data collection and analysis were performed by Danapriya Visvanathan. Danapriya Visvanathan wrote the first draft of the manuscript, and all authors commented on previous versions of the manuscript. All authors read and approved the final manuscript.

REFERENCES

[1]   D.J.   Cennimo,   "What   is   COVID-19?",   **2021**.   Available   at: https://www.medscape.com/answers/2500114-197401/what-is-COVID-19(Accessed on: 4th August 2021).

[2]   "Coronavirus   disease   (COVID-19)",   **2022**.   Available   at: https://www.who.int/health-

topics/coronavirus#tab=tab_1 (Accessed on: 6th June 2021).

[3]   K. Pearce, "What is social distancing and how can it slow the spread of COVID-19?", **2022**. Available at: https://hub.jhu.edu/2020/03/13/what-is-social- distancing/ (Accessed on: 8th June 2021).

[4]   H. H. Goh, "The importance of social distancing during a pandemic", Available at: https://www.nst.com.my/opinion/columnists/2020/03/578050/importance- (Accessed on: 10th June 2021).

[5]   R. Sarah, "What is Social Distancing and Why is it Important?", Available at: https://healthtalk.unchealthcare.org/what-is-social-distancing-and-why-is-it- important/ (Accessed on: 15th June 2021).

[6]   Z. Shah, D. Surian, A. Dyda, E. Coiera, K.D. Mandl, and A.G. Dunn, "Automatically appraising the credibility of vaccine-related web pages shared on social media", *A Twitter Surveillance Study,* vol. 21, no. 11, p. 2, 2019.
[http://dx.doi.org/10.2196/14007]

[7]   A. Wong, S. Ho, O. Olusanya, M.V. Antonini, and D. Lyness, "The use of social media and online communications in times of pandemic COVID-19,", vol. 22, no. 3, pp. 255-260, Oct. **2020**.

[8]   L. Li, A. Aldosery, F. Vitiugin, N. Nathan, D.N. Ortiz, C. Castillo, and P. Kostkova, "The response of governments and public health agencies to COVID-19 pandemics on social media", *A Multi-Country Analysis of Twitter Discourse,* pp. 1-4, 2021.
[http://dx.doi.org/10.3389/fpubh.2021.716333]

[9]   E. Merkley, A. Bridgman, P.J. Loewen, T. Owen, D. Ruths, and O. Zhilin, "A rare moment of cross-partisan consensus: elite and public response to the COVID-19 pandemic in canada"", *Canadian Journal of Political Scien,* vol. 53, no. 2, pp. 311-318, 2020.
[http://dx.doi.org/10.1017/S0008423920000311]

[10]   Y. Wang, H. Hao, and L.S. Platt, "Examining risk and crisis communications of government agencies and stakeholders during early-stages of COVID-19 on twitter", *Computers in Human Behavior,* pp. 1-25, 2020.
[http://dx.doi.org/10.1016/j.chb.2020.106568]

[11]   C.H. Basch, G.C. Hillyer, Z.C.M. Erwin, C. Jaime, J. Mohlman, and C.E. Basch, "Preventive Behaviors Conveyed on YouTube to Mitigate Transmission of COVID-19: Cross-Sectional Study", *JMIR Public Health and Surveillance,* vol. 6, no. 2, p. e18807, 2020.
[http://dx.doi.org/10.2196/18807]

[12]   D. Chaffey, "Global social media research summary", **2021**. Available at: https://www.smartinsights.com/social-media-marketing/social-media-strategy/new- global-socia--media-research/(Accessed on: 7th June, 2021).

[13]   E. Ferrara, "COVID-19 on Twitter: Bots, Conspiracies, and Social Media Activism", April 2020",

[14]   M. Saud, M. Mashud, and R. Ida, "Usage of social media during the pandemic: Seeking support and awareness about COVID-19 through social media platforms,", *Journal of Public Affairs,* vol. 20, no. 4, pp. 1-14, September 2020.
[http://dx.doi.org/10.1002/pa.2417]

[15]   E. Dong, H. Du, and L. Gardner, "An interactive web-based dashboard to track COVID-19 in real time,", *The Lancet Infectious Diseases,* vol. 20, no. 5, pp. 533-534, February 2020.
[http://dx.doi.org/10.1016/S1473-3099(20)30120-1]

[16]   V. Trifonova, "How the outbreak has changed the way we use social media", **2020**. Available at: https://blog.gwi.com/chart-of-the-week/social-media-amid-the-outbreak/(Accessed on: 29th June, 2021).

[17]   S. Wold, Available at: COVID-19 is changing how, why and how much we're using social media para. 2-4, Sept. 16, **2020**.https://www.digitalcommerce360.com/2020/09/16/COVID-19-is-changing-how-why-and-how-much-were-using-social-media/(Accessed on: 25th June, 2021).

[18]   "Importance of Social Media Marketing During COVID-19", Palgrave Macmillan, **2021**.

[19]   H. Susanto, L.F.F. Yie, and F. Mohiddin, "Revealing Social Media Phenomenon in Time of COVID-19 Pandemic for Boosting Start-Up Businesses through Digital Ecosystem,", *Applied System Innovation,* vol. 4, no. 6, pp. 2-21, 2021.
[http://dx.doi.org/10.3390/asi4010006]

[20]   Kirdaglig, "What are the benefits of using social media during the coronavirus pandemic?", Broomfield   School,   para.   2-4,   June   7,   **2020**.   Available   at: https://www.broomfield.enfield.sch.uk/post/advantages-
of-social-media-during-the-coronavirus-pandemic(Accessed on: 12th June, 2021).

[21]   D.A.G. Padilla, and L.T. Blanco, ""Social media influence in the COVID-19 Pandemic," International braz j urol: vol. 46", *official journal of the Brazilian Society of Urology,* pp. 1-4.
[http://dx.doi.org/10.1590/S1677-5538]

[22]   J. Abbas, D. Wang, Z. Su, and A. Ziapour, "The Role of Social Media in the Advent of COVID-19 Pandemic: Crisis Management, Mental Health Challenges and Implications,", *Risk Manag Healthc Policy,* vol. 14, pp. 1917-1932, 2021.
[http://dx.doi.org/10.2147/RMHP.S284313]

[23]   A.K.M. Chan, C.P. Nickson, J.W. Rudolph, A. Lee, and G.M. Joynt, "Social media for rapid knowledge dissemination: early experience from the COVID-19 pandemic", *Association of Anaesthetists,* vol. 75, no. 12, pp. 1579-1582, 2020.
[http://dx.doi.org/10.1111/anae.15057]

[24]   M. Samy, R. Abdelmalak, A. Ahmed, and M. Kelada, "Social media as a source of medical information during COVID-19", *Medical Education Online,* vol. 25, no. 1, 2020.
[http://dx.doi.org/10.1080/10872981.2020.1791467]

[25]   W. Sawahel, "Social media offers platform for online learning – Study", Available at: https://www.universityworldnews.com/post.php?story=20200909144604255(Accessed on: 14th June, 2021).

[26]   C. Greenhow, and C. Lewin, "Social media and education: Reconceptualizing the boundaries of formal and informal learning,", *Learning Media and Technology,* vol. 41, pp. 1-25, 2021.

[27]   V. Balakrishnan, and C.L. Gan, "Students' learning styles and their effects on the use of social media technology for learning", *Telematics and Informatics,* vol. 33, no. 3, pp. 808-821, 2016.
[http://dx.doi.org/10.1016/j.tele.2015.12.004]

[28]   T. Gonulal, "The Use of Instagram as a Mobile-Assisted Language Learning Tool", *Contemporary Educational Technology,* vol. 10, no. 3, pp. 309-323, 2019.
[http://dx.doi.org/10.30935/cet.590108]

[29]   T.M. Khan, "Use of social media and WhatsApp to conduct teaching activities during the COVID-19 lockdown in Pakistan", *International Journal of Pharmacy Practice,* vol. 29, no. 1, p. 90, 2020.
[http://dx.doi.org/10.1111/ijpp.12659]

[30]   P. Suciu, "During COVID-19 Outbreak Can YouTube Help Keep Students Engaged?", Available at: https://www.forbes.com/sites/petersuciu/2020/04/09/during-COVID-19-outbreak-can-youtub-
-help-keep-students-engaged/?sh=78b631f078de(Accessed on: 5th July, 2021).

[31]   Z. Yaacob, and N.H.M. Saad, "Acceptance of YouTube as a Learning Platform during the COVID-19 Pandemic: The Moderating Effect of Subscription Status", *TEM Journal,* vol. 9, no. 4, pp. 1732-1739, 2020.
[http://dx.doi.org/10.18421/TEM94-54]

[32]   M. Iqbal, S. Latifah, and I. Irwandani, "Channel Youtube Video Blog (Vlog) Development With Stem Approach As An Alternative Learning Media", *Inovasi Pembangunan : Jurnal Kelitbangan,* vol. 7, no. 2, p. 135, 2019.

[33]   N.L.D.S. Dewi, and N.P.S.E. Carniasih, "The Influence of Youtube-based Learning Media in English Grammar Learning", *Faculty of Economics and Humanities,* pp. 397-403, 2018.
[http://dx.doi.org/10.24071/ijiet.v7i1.5315]

[34]   N. Azlan, S. Zakaria, and M. Yunus, "WhatsApp Messenger as a Learning Tool: An Investigation of Pre-service Teachers' Learning without Instructor Presence,", *International Journal of Academic Research in Business and Social Sciences,* vol. 9, pp. 620-636, 2019.

[35]   S.S. Shazali, Z.H. Shamsudin, and M.M. Yunus, "Instagram: A Platform to Develop Student's Writing Ability", *International Journal of Academic Research in Business and Social Sciences,* vol. 9, pp. 88-98, 2019.
[http://dx.doi.org/10.6007/IJARBSS/v9-i1/5365]

[36]   U. Supiandi, S. Sari, and C. Subarkah, "Enhancing Students Higher Order Thinking Skill through Instagram based Flipped Classroom Learning Model,", *Atlantis Press,* pp. 233-237, 2019.
[http://dx.doi.org/10.2991/aes-18.2019.55]

[37]   M. Manaroinsong, "The use of instagram as mobile learning to support english cognitive learning process", *Faculty of psychology and socio-cultural sciences islamic university of indonesia,* pp. 8-9, 2018.

[38]   Susanti Susanti, "The Use of WhatsApp in Reading Lesson at the STMIK Pontianak, West Kalimantan, Indonesia", *MIMBAR PENDIDIKAN: Jurnal Indonesia untuk Kajian Pendidikan,* vol. 5, no. 1, pp. 58-62, 2020.

[39]   A. Alenazi, "WhatsApp Messenger as a Learning Tool: An Investigation of Pre-service Teachers' Learning without Instructor Presence", *Journal of Education and Training Studies,* vol. 6, no. 1, 2018.
[http://dx.doi.org/10.11114/jets.v6i1.2684]

[40]   Kang Kang, and W. Chen, "Art in the Age of Social Media: Interaction Behavior Analysis of Instagram Art Accounts", *Informatics,* vol. 6, no. 4, p. 52, 2019.
[http://dx.doi.org/10.3390/informatics6040052]

[41]   J. Kushner, "The role of social media during a pandemic", para. 5-9, March 25, **2020**. Available at: https://khoros.com/blog/social-medias-role-during-COVID-19(Accessed on: 21st June, 2021).

[42]   S. Izmailova, "25 Online Fundraising Ideas Perfect for Any Cause (Social Distancing Approved!)", Available at: https://www.wildapricot.com/blog/online-fundraising(Accessed on: 27th June, 2021).

[43]   M. Fornillos, "COVID's impact on social media marketing—& what you can do about it", **2021**. Available   at: https://www.agilitypr.com/pr-news/public-relations/covids-impact-on-social-media-marketing-and-what-you-can-do-about-it/(Accessed on: 15th July, 2021).

[44]   E.   Pacheco,   "COVID-19's   Impact   on   Social   Media   Usage",   **2020**.   Available   at: https://www.thebrandonagency.com/blog/COVID-19s-impact-on-social-media-usage/(Accessed on: 16th July, 2021).

[45]   G. Henderson, "5 Ways to Use Social Media for Connection During Times of Social Distancing", Available at: https://www.searchenginejournal.com/5-ways-to-use- social-media-for-connect-on-during-times-of-social-distancing/358080/#close(Accessed on: 14th July, 2021).

CHAPTER 6

AI based Clinical Analysis of COVID-19 Infected Patients

Mohamed Yousuff[1,*], Rajasekhara Babu[1], R. Anusha[1] and M.A. Matheen[1]

[1] *School of Computer Science and Engineering, Vellore Institute of Technology, Vellore, Tamil Nadu, India*

Abstract: Severe Acute Respiratory Syndrome Coronavirus 2 (SARS-CoV-2) is an unknown beta coronavirus that comes under the B genus, which causes Coronavirus Disease 2019 (COVID-19), a declared universal epidemic, posing a serious menace to human health irrespective of the nationality. According to the World Health Organization (WHO) statistics, as of September 10, 2021, there were 223,022,539 positive cases of COVID-19 with 4,602,883 fatalities reported worldwide. A total of 5,352,927,297 vaccine doses have been facilitated since September 5, 2021. This pandemic has become a ravaging illness because of its highly contractible nature and mutations. Many types of research in diverse fields of science have been initiated to suppress the effects and manage the havoc. Artificial Intelligence (AI) is classified as a subdomain of science, which most certainly contributed to numerous applications in confronting the present state at a broader level. In this chapter, we have tried to explore state-of-the-art AI techniques implemented in the perspective of COVID-19 across multiple subjects of concern. The AI approaches are utilized in the treatment, diagnosis, prediction of recovery, severity and mortality of patients, chest X-Ray and computed tomography-based analysis, pandemic prediction, its control and management, pharmaceutical research, COVID-19 text corpus processing, and virus apprehension. Thus, the comprehension of various applications is meant to enlighten the status of AI in this pandemonium. Finally, we conclude with some suggestions and remarks to tackle the disaster in an improved way.

Keywords: SARS-CoV-2, Artificial intelligence, Machine learning, Deep learning, COVID-19 treatment, COVID-19 diagnostics, Mobile application, COVID-19 text processing, COVID-19 recovery, COVID-19 mortality, COVID-19 disease severity, Forecasting AI-models, COVID-19 risk evaluation, COVID-19 safety measures, COVID-19 false information, Pandemic energy services, COVID-19 drug repositioning, COVID-19 immune system analysis, COVID-19 vaccine development, COVID-19 contagion pathogen.

---

[*] **Corresponding author Mohamed Yousuff:** School of Computer Science and Engineering, Vellore Institute of Technology, Vellore, Tamil Nadu, India; Tel: +813049281; E-mail: yousuffrashid@gmail.com

INTRODUCTION

COVID-19 is an exceptional disorder caused by a deadly pathogen named SARS-CoV-2. An initial confirmed case was discovered by the end of December 2019 in the Wuhan region, China. Subsequently, the infection has disseminated swiftly, resulting in a pandemic [1]. According to World Health Organization (WHO) statistics, as of September 10, 2021, there were 223,022,539 positive cases of COVID-19, with 4,602,883 fatalities reported worldwide. A total of 5,352,927,297 vaccine doses had been facilitated since September 5, 2021 [2]. The flu-like signs of the disease include coughing, fever, exhaustion, breathlessness, lack of odor and appetite, migraine, and muscle discomfort are the common indications of the infection [1].

The virus's primary genesis is still unknown, but investigations on the virus's genome sequence have revealed that it belongs to the β-CoV genus under coronavirus species originating from mammal hosts, more specifically bats and rodents. SARS-CoV-2 spreads *via* direct touch and air. It enters respiratory cells by bonding to "Angiotensin-Converting Enzyme 2 (ACE2)". As the virus mutates, it causes numerous issues in all aspects of human existence, and new challenges arise as time passes. Each day, advanced innovations are designed to tackle these quickly increasing difficulties [3].

The exploration and implementation of technologies that mimic human intellect are called Artificial Intelligence (AI). AI is proving itself as an effective technology in a broad spectrum of sectors, notably hoax detection, computer vision, digital advertising, robotics, and autonomous driving vehicles, and so on. With its achievements in fields such as the diagnosis of diseases, medication, patient observation, drug development, epidemiology, and so on, there is a great aspiration that AI will become a flourishing field of research to address the difficulties that humanity is currently experiencing [4].

It is believed that AI will be critical in aiding medical and academic research on COVID-19 and subsequent events. For example, at the start of the pandemic, China implemented a series of anti-virus measures, including using AI-based technology. In this endeavor, they investigated using facial recognition sensors to detect diseased individuals, drones to sanitize spaces, bots to transport food and medicines, *etc* [5]. Constituent elements of AI are depicted in Fig. (**1**).

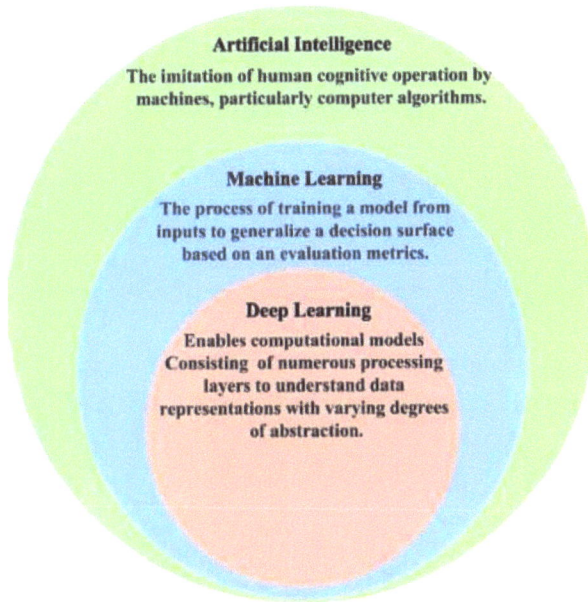

Artificial Intelligence

The imitation of human cognitive operation by machines, particularly computer algorithms.

Machine Learning

The process of training a model from inputs to generalize a decision surface based on an evaluation metrics.

Deep Learning

Enables computational models Consisting of numerous processing layers to understand data representations with varying degrees of abstraction.

Fig. (1). Relationship between AI, ML and DL.

Machine Learning (ML)

ML is a data analysis technique that facilitates the creation of analytical models. It is a subfield of AI predicated on the premise that algorithms can learn from data inputs, spot patterns, and decide things with little or no human interference. Increasing data quantities and variety, cost-effective, more efficient computing and processing, and low-cost data storage are the motivating factors for ML evolution. Hence, the models can be created rapidly and autonomously to evaluate larger, more complicated information and offer faster, more precise results, even on a massive scale. An organization improves its chances of recognizing valuable possibilities or avoiding unexpected risks by developing detailed models [6].

ML is broadly classified into five subsections, as shown in Fig. **2** This chapter. mainly involves supervised, unsupervised, and DL. A dependent variable in statistics is referred to as a label in ML. Similarly, a variable in statistics is referred to as a feature in ML. The ML algorithm is trained using a set of features and their corresponding labels to predict the label of new features. The process of categorizing a given dataset into class labels is known as classification. For example, discriminating between cancer and normal data points. Logistic Regression (LR), Naïve Bayes (NB), Stochastic Gradient Descent (SGD), K-Nearest Neighbors (KNN), Decision Tree (DT), Random Forest (RF), Support Vector Machine (SVM) and Multi-Layer Perceptron (MLP) or Artificial Neural Networks (ANN) are most commonly used classification algorithms. Accuracy

(Ă), Sensitivity (Ŝ), Specificity (Ş), Precision, Recall, and F1-score are the popular performance measures for the classification task.

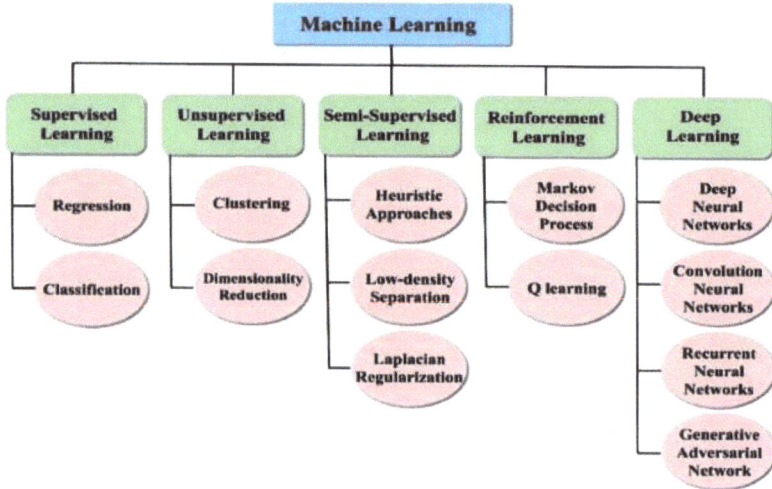

Fig. (2). Types of ML techniques.

The regression technique represents the association between a target and single or multiple predictors (independent) values. Regression analysis, in particular, enables us to comprehend how the value of the target variable transforms into predictor variable(s). In contrast, some of the predictor variables are maintained constant. It forecasts the real values like lifespan, income, cost, temperature *etc*. Linear Regression (LinReg), Logistic Regression (LR), Polynomial Regression (PR), Support Vector Regression (SVR), and Decision Tree Regression (DTR), Random Forest Regression (RFR), Ridge Regression (RR), and Lasso Regression (LasReg) are most widely used regression algorithms. Mean Squared Error (MSE), Root Mean Squared Error (RMSE), Mean Absolute Error (MAE), and Area Under the ROC Curve (AUC) are the established metrics for regression tasks.

Clustering is an approach that groups observations in the dataset (data point) together. The clustering method is used to classify each data point in a specific class. Data points in the same cluster are expected to have comparable traits and attributes, whereas data points in other clusters exhibit wildly divergent qualities. K-Means, Density-Based Spatial Clustering of Applications with Noise (DBSCAN), and Hierarchical Agglomerative clustering are some eminent clustering techniques. When a dataset consists of an enormous number of features for each observation or data point, then the Dimensionality Reduction approach is used to transform high dimensional data into a low dimension or latent space to ensure high-performance metrics.

Deep Learning (DL)

DL, a well-known subset of ML that employs numerous layers to excerpt relatively significant properties from raw input. In image processing, for example, lower layers could recognize boundaries, while upper layers could discover features meaningful to humans, like numerals, characters, or faces. The term "deep" represents several data transforming layers. DL model structures can be built using a biased layer-by-layer approach. DL assists in disentangling this generalization and determining which aspects increase performance. Specific varieties of neural networks (NN) exist, but they all share the same elements: neurons, activation function, weight, and bias term. These elements behave similarly to biological neurons and are trained in the same way as ML algorithms [7]. Deep Neural Networks (DNN), Convolution Neural Networks, (CNN) and Recurrent Neural Networks (RNN) are the subcategories of NN with more implementations in the context of this chapter.

DNNs are generally Feedforward Neural Networks (FNN) in which data moves toward the destination output layer from the initial input layer without circling backward. Initially, the DNN constructs a mapping of units called virtual neurons and gives arbitrary integer values termed as weights to the linkages connecting them. The weights, inputs, and sometimes bias values are multiplied, yielding a value range of 0 and 1. If the model failed to perceive a specific pattern, then the algorithm would alter the values of weights using the backpropagation learning technique. As a result, the algorithm can increase the importance of specific features until it identifies the precise mathematical operation to analyze the data thoroughly. The architecture of DNN is shown in Fig. (**3**).

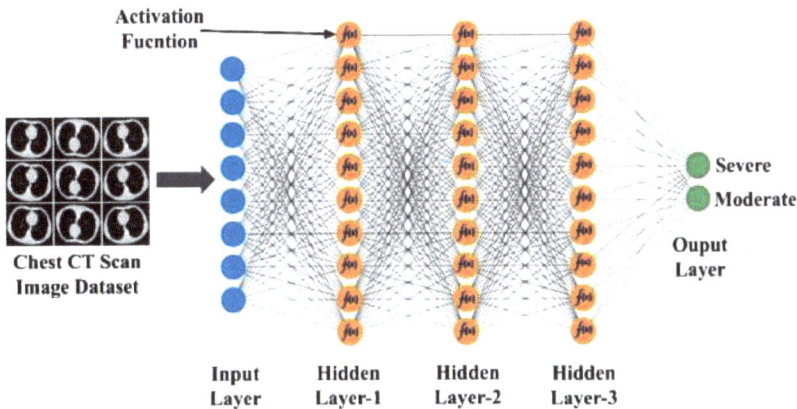

Fig. (3). DNN architecture to classify medical images based on the severity of the disease.

CNNs are typically used to evaluate visual information. They are also termed shift-invariant because they use kernel or filter sliding to extract the features from the input images. Biological mechanisms motivated the development of CNN. Any intermediary layers in an FNN are referred to as hidden since their input features and output values are concealed by the activation function. Typically, CNN comprises a convolution layer that performs the dot product computation tasks between the kernel and the input data matrix. It is often the Frobenius multiplication and generally uses Rectified Linear Unit (ReLU) as an activation function.

The convolution procedure produces a feature map, which feeds the data to the following layer. Additional layers like pooling layers, Fully Connected Layers (FCL), dropout layers for regularization (avoids over-fitting), and batch normalization layers are added. Pooling layers minimize the dimensionality of data. Finally, to determine the input images, the flattened matrix is passed through an FCL [7]. A general CNN architecture is depicted in Fig. (4).

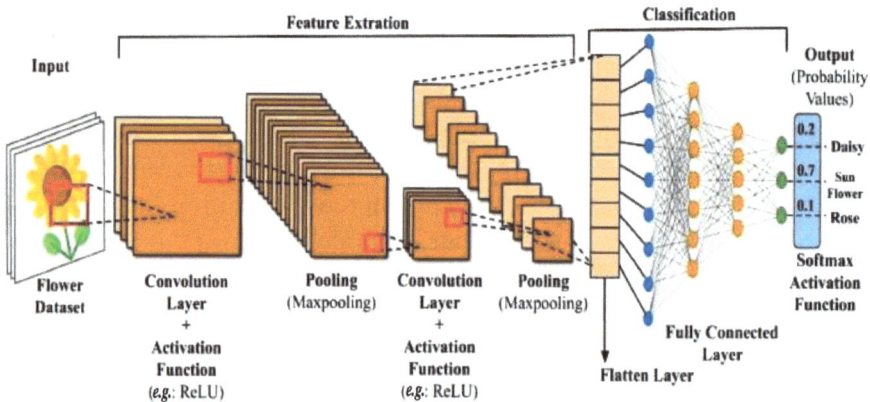

Fig. (4). General CNN architecture to classify the different categorizes of flower.

In RNN, unit interconnections form a directed graph with time series. As a result, it can reveal periodic vibrant characteristics. RNNs have evolved from FNN and can process changeable length series of inputs using their state space (memory). The phrase RNN refers to two major kinds of NN with a similar overall design; one is termed a finite impulse, and the second is known as an infinite impulse. Both impulses are using additional stored states. If the memory includes latency or feedback mechanisms, it can be substituted with another structure or graph. These regulated states are known as gated memory; and are used in Long Short-Term Memory (LSTM) networks.

Physically extracting characteristics from an image necessitates a thorough understanding of the specific topic and the domain. The feature extraction process takes a lot of time, so developing an ML model is affected by the time factor, but with the help of DL this procedure is automated. Fig. (**5**) and Table **1** depict the difference between ML and DL.s

Table 1. Distinction between ML and DL algorithms.

Constraints	ML	DL
Information requirement	It is comfortably feasible to train on less data.	It demands a huge amount of data.
Performance	Comparatively less accuracy	Ensures high accuracy metric.
Model training	Faster training time	Consumes lot of time during training phase.
Dependencies	Central processing unit are sufficient for execution.	Requires graphical processing unit for faster execution.
Hyperparameter tuning	Capabilities for tuning is limited	Promotes broader spectrum of ways to tune.

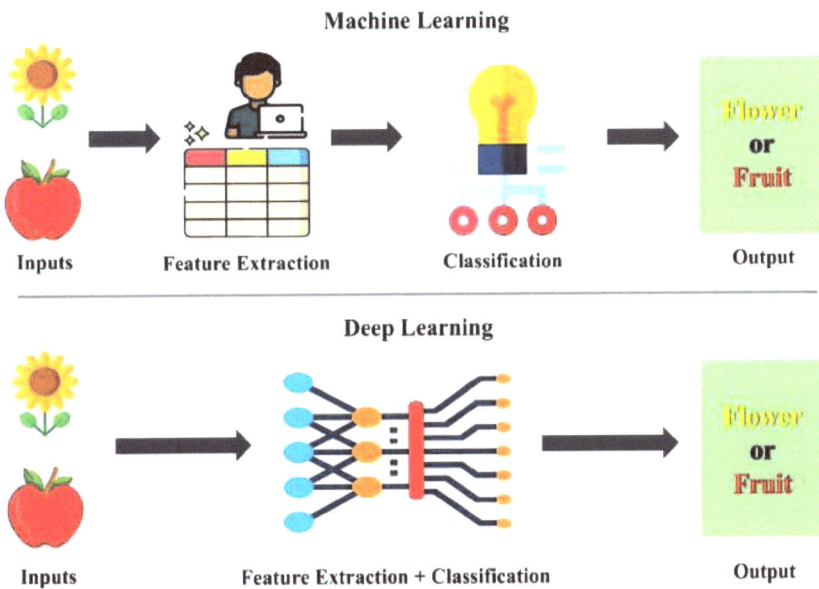

Fig. (5). Difference between ML and DL while performing an image classification task.

The chapter is well-ordered in the following structure; section **2** elaborates on the utilization of AI in clinical applications. Section **3** depicts AI implementations in addressing and resolving epidemiology problems. Section **4,** explain the utilization of AI-based techniques in the pharmaceutical domain. Section **5** details the AI approaches that helped to understand the virus. Finally, the chapter is completed in section **6** with appropriate remarks for future research.

CLINICAL APPLICATIONS

This section of the chapter discusses the medical and clinical implications of AI techniques for the medicament of COVID-19 victims.

Treatment

A significant domain of implementing AI in handling the COVID-19 outbreak is the methodologies intended to treat the pandemic. There exists a complexity for professionals and laypersons to determine the resemblance instantly and precisely and disparities between the diverse mutations and target the salient features of the novel mutation. An intelligent analysis approach based on ML can instinctively inspect the resemblance and disparities of distinct medicament plans, communicate the emphasis of the unusual mutation to physicians, and minimize the level of complication in understanding the "diagnosis and treatment plan" for the clinicians and the ordinary people. Empirical results ($Ă = 100\%$) indicate that AI-based techniques can accurately predict and equate the novel variant of the program text's topic in an unsupervised manner to an existing variant of the program's text [8].

In the initial phases of the epidemic, AI models are necessary for predicting the necessity for oxygen therapeutics. The AI model trained with combined features from clinical metadata and radiography images performed better in predicting the need for oxygen therapeutics with the highest metric ($Ă=95\%$). Although the ML model has comparatively lesser accuracy than the multimodal DL modal, it persisted adequately perfect for clinical triage under the pandemic situations [9]. One issue in treating patients is the equipment limitations, such as ventilator systems. In such circumstances, hospitals are frequently confronted with the critical decision of which patient is preferred to receive such care. An AI-based decision-making algorithm, which works in a three-phase approach, is suggested to resolve the prioritization problem. The first phase results in a determination matrix computed on infected patient list convergence and biological laboratory test criteria. The second phase involves weighing the test criteria by respiratory domain specialists. The third phase gives the final patient priorities in individual and group contexts [10].

The recovered individuals who recently suffered from declining COVID-19 infection have a definite chance of having antibodies circulating in their bloodstream. Strengthening the immune system is the key to fighting the host viruses, which can be achieved by transfusion of antibodies from recovered persons to currently deteriorating patients. Anatomically, dual confrontations must overcome and permit recuperating plasma transfusion to save acute COVID-19 individuals. Primarily, recovering individuals should satisfy donor selection plasma constrain and obey the national health organization's standards, terms, and procedures. Secondly, critical decision-making is involved in selecting the most appropriate recuperating plasma and prioritizing infected patients. ML algorithms play a vital role in identifying the best suitable recuperating plasma for the most crucial patients [11].

Diagnostics

Many official authorities, including the WHO, feel that testing is vital in managing the pandemic because it provides pertinent data about smaller outbreaks that may control before they escalate. The present testing methodology is "Reverse Transcription Polymerase Chain Reaction (RT-PCR)" with determining the nucleotide sequences and recognition. RT-PCR consumes a lot of resources, time and is relatively expensive. There have also been tests developed using IgM/IgG antibodies. However, their sensitivity ($\hat{S}$) and specificity ($Ş$) are limited. To obtain the best outcomes, accurately diagnosing the clinical level of COVID-19 patients is critical. Currently, patients are classified as serious or non-serious based on a few clinical characteristics that do not adequately define the disease's complex pathological, physiological, and immunological reaction. AI approaches have been utilized in certain studies to identify illness without needing radiography images and RT-PCR.

ML techniques are used with data from 151 published research to develop a fair and precise diagnostic model for the illness based on COVID-19 symptoms and regular testing results. The study establishes a link between being male and having more significant serum lymphocyte and neutrophil counts. Accordingly, individuals with COVID-19 may be grouped into subgroups based on their serum immune cell levels, disease indications, and sex. XGBoost algorithm is deployed, and a $\hat{S}$ of 93% and a $Ş$ of 98% are reported [12]. The data collected from patients undergoing hemodialysis due to renal failure is trained on an ML model to forecast the likelihood of individuals possessing an undiagnosed COVID-19 contagion [13]. An AI system is presented for diagnosing pandemic cases based on radiography images, clinical symptoms, exposure history, and laboratory tests of 905 individuals, 419 of whom are proven to be COVID-19 positive in the laboratory [14].

Brazil takes the lead in COVID-19 cases among the other South American countries. Nonetheless, underdiagnosis is widespread in the nation. Applying nowcasting techniques in combination with ML approaches can aid in estimating the number of new instances of the illness. Recent advancements in ML techniques provide the potential for nowcasting refinement. The ML technique categorizes instances that have not yet received a diagnosis, resulting in the nowcast. To assess underdiagnosis, the variation noted in the absence of nowcasting, and the median of the nowcasting predictions is compared for the whole period [15]. An Ensemble of ML algorithms such as LR, SVM, DT and RF has been utilized to diagnose the illness [16].

DL Models

To expedite the medication and diagnostics of SARS-CoV-2 illness, several DL techniques are used, especially Long Short-Term Memory (LSTMs), Extreme Learning Machines (ELMs), and Generative Adversarial Networks (GANs). According to researchers, these techniques can assemble a continuity of unstructured and structured data inputs. A Deep Neural Network (DNN) method is combined with ML techniques to monitor patients and provide enhanced curation. CovidDeep is a platform that affiliates a DNN with habiliment remedial sensors to facilitate widespread viral and ailment testing. The model is not trained on features that are extracted manually; instead depends on features accumulated from a habiliment device and a few simply answerable questionnaire queries [17, 18].

Diagnostics via Blood Tests

Physicians caring for COVID-19 patients have observed a variety of alterations in regular blood values. These alterations, however, preclude them from conducting COVID-19 diagnosis. An ML model for the diagnosis of COVID-19 was developed and cross-validated using standard blood tests from patients with a variety of bacterial and viral illnesses, as well as COVID-19-positive patients. According to the XGBoost algorithm's feature significance score, the list of most effective regular blood indicators for COVID-19 diagnostics are as follows; "eosinophil ratio, prothrombin activity percentage, mean corpuscular hemoglobin concentration and prothrombin international normalized ratio." The observed diagnostic accuracy is equivalent to, if not superior to, that of RT-PCR and chest CT investigations [19].

An approach based on AI is devised to conduct an initial checking of suspicious SARS-CoV-2 patients entering the ultimate healthcare section. An ML classifier uses commonly available primary blood test data to classify samples as positive (infected with SARS-CoV-2) or cynical (disinfected). Positive patients can be sent for additional confirmatory testing *(e.g.,* radiography images or distinct immunoglobulins). This study uses data from 5,644 patients made publicly available by Brazil's Albert Einstein Hospital. A sample of 600 persons, including

82 SARS-CoV-2 infected individuals, are considered. Utilizing the sampled dataset, an AI classification system is developed to determine whether doubtful patients admitted to the emergency cabin were likely to be virus negative. Patients anticipated as positive by the framework should be instantly isolated from others while confirmatory tests are in progress. Thus, assisting in minimizing the spread of further infections [20].

Enhancing DNA Tests

RT-PCR with virus DNA detection remains the gold standard for COVID-19 diagnosis. In a pseudo-convolutional technique, the DNA sequences are broken down into smaller segments and sequences with overlap and expressed by co-occurrence matrices. The analysis is performed on the obtained nucleotide acquired using the RT-PCR approach, obviating the need for sequence alignment. This approach enables the identification of virus genomes from a vast library (currently 348,364 pathogen genomes), belonging to 25 virus genus including SARS-Cov-2. A real-world resemblance analysis of SARS-Cov-2 to Coronaviridae and disinfected person genome, performance measures $\hat{S}$=98% and $\check{S}$=99% using MLP. Thus, the infinitesimal diagnostics of SARS-CoV-2 can be improved by integrating RT-PCR with the pseudo-convolutional technique to recognize SARS-Cov-2 DNA sequences rapidly and accurately [21].

AI-based Mobile Applications

The incompetence to test at a broader range is still a challenge and fatal weakness in the ceaseless battle against the pandemic. Quantifiable checking equipment would be a turning point. "AI4COVID-19" is an AI-powered smartphone app developed based on previous methodologies on cough-based analysis of respiratory sickness. It is deployed as a mobile app and utilized as a screening solution for COVID-19 contagion. The mobile application captured and forwards the cough audio (30 Deci seconds) to an intelligent processing unit powered by AI and operated on the cloud, delivering the decision in no time. Coughing is an indication of over 35 different medical diseases that are unrelated to COVID-19. This complicates the multidisciplinary task of diagnosing a COVID-19 infection solely by coughing. This issue is dealt with by examining the unusual morphologic variations caused by SARS-CoV-2 pathological conditions in the lungs compared to those caused by other respiratory illnesses [22].

Transfer learning is used to manage limited cough samples data available for training. The results indicate that "AI4COVID-19" can discriminate between SARS-CoV-2 inflicted coughs and numerous non-SARS-CoV-2 inflicted coughs. The performance metrics are remarkable to justify a vast accumulation of clearly labeled cough observations to assess "AI4COVID-19's" generalizability. It is not a diagnostic tool of clinical quality. Rather than that, it provides a screening tool that can be used anytime, anyplace, and by anybody. Additionally, it can be utilized as a medical situation determination tool to direct clinical diagnosis and counseling for individuals in most need, ultimately rescuing many lives [22].

COVID-19 Text Corpus Processing

The standard and ensemble ML algorithms are utilized to perform the classification task on text corpus (clinical reports) to discriminate them into four classes. Features vectors are generated with the help of feature engineering approaches, namely "Bag of words (BOW) and Term frequency/inverse document frequency (TF/IDF)." The obtained feature vectors are fed into the conventional and ensemble ML classifiers. LR and Multinomial Naive Bayes (NB) models excelled with an accuracy of 96.2% on testing data compared to other ML models. The text data is amassed *via* an online questionnaire. This preprocessed text corpus is subjected to various prediction techniques, including LR, SVM, and MLP. Based on COVID-19 signs and symptoms, these algorithms are used to predict prospective SARS-CoV-2 patients. MLP demonstrated the highest accuracy (91.62%) compared to the other models. Likewise, the SVM demonstrated the highest precision (92%) [23, 24].

Inspecting Infected Individuals

It is a challenge in healthcare units and clinics to inspect the state of SARS-CoV-2 infected patients without exposing frontline health personnel to the virus. This section discusses the applications of AI in patient monitoring and prediction.

Predicting Recovery and Mortality

Due to resource constraints, hospitals may be unable to give all patients with severe symptoms the necessary observation, diagnosis, and treatment. Predicting a patient's recuperation or fatality rate is critical in this regard, as this knowledge can assist hospitals in allocating medical resources more proficiently.

Classification of data acquired between February 19, 2020, and March 21, 2020, is utilized by the ANN approach. Seven distinct variables, namely group, contagion reason, gender, confirmation date, year of birth, country, and region, are used to train the classifier. The neural network model examines the most significant variables in cured and fatal cases. The findings indicated that the predictive classifier could accurately predict survived and died instances. Additionally, it is discovered that determining the cause of the infection increases the likelihood that the patient is recovered. This suggests that the virus may be controllable based on the transmission source. Furthermore, earlier detection of the condition enables good control and a greater chance of recovery [25].

The supervised ML techniques are intended to discover risk factors linked with death in COVID-19 individuals. Medical data of 1086 COVID-19 cases are accumulated from the online data scientist community (Kaggle) from January 12, 2020, to February 28, 2020. Finally, the RF classification technique use a sample dataset of 430 cases to discover significant predictors and their impact on fatality. During model validation on the test data, the AUC was 0.97. The main predictor of death was age, preceded by the time interval between symptom start and admission to the hospital. Patients over the age of 62 had a greater risk of death; however, appropriate medication and care within two days of the beginning of signs have been shown to decrease death rates in COVID-19 patients [26].

Conducting a rapid, reliable, and prompt clinical evaluation of the disease severity is vital. To aid in decision-making and operational strategy in health services, a repository of blood samples from 485 affected individuals in the Wuhan area of China is being investigated to identify critical predictive indicators of mortality rate. For this objective, ML technologies identified three biomarkers that accurately forecast the fatality rate of each patient with 90% accuracy around two weeks in advance [27]. An ML-based prediction model is also used to detect patients at risk of impending Intensive Care Unit (ICU) transfer within 24 hours; this approach, can significantly improve hospital resource utilization and patient flow scheduling [28]. An open-source ML tool called CoCoMoRP is developed using publicly accessible surveillance data for providing better care to people hospitalized with COVID-19 by assessing the danger of mortality amongst COVID-19-positive persons [29].

Predicting the Level of Disease Severity

Individuals with SARS-CoV-2 infection typically exhibit serious symptoms, and some people with acute conditions even die or experience catastrophic organ damage. As a result, the objective has been to forecast the severity of symptoms.

A method that can accurately identify severe COVID-19 and assist in medical decision-making for COVID-19 patients is urgently needed. 590 COVID-19 hospitalized patients are considered (training set = 285; validation set = 127; test set = 178). After filtering the training set using two ML methods, five out of thirty-one medical features are included in the model training phase to compute the likelihood of getting intense COVID-19 illness [30]. Graph Neural Networks (GNN) is widely used to excerpt substantial depictions from graph-organized data and to accomplish forecasting activities like node categorization and link determination. A methodology is described for generating new edge features in

GNNs using an integration of ML, which is eventually implemented to perform node categorization problems. This technique forecasts infection and severity in COVID-19 individuals [31].

COVID-19 patients with consistently moderate sickness admitted to Wuhan Pulmonary Hospital between January 2, 2020, and February 14, 2020, are classified into two sections: those who progressed to malignancy and those who did not. The predictive models are built using multivariate LR and DL approaches, and their AUC metrics are compared. DL algorithms could exactly and effectively detect mild patients who are prone to degenerate into severe or critical cases, which undoubtedly aids in optimizing treatment strategies, reducing fatality rate, and relieving medication and treatment stress [32]. The COVID-19 severity identification model is constructed using ML algorithms. Thirty three features are determined as being strongly linked with COVID-19 severity; an SVM model displayed a promising identification accuracy. Moreover, these 33 features are subjected to redundancy checks. The final SVM model is trained upon 29 features and attained a metric Ã=81%. This approach could aid in the risk assessment of COVID-19 individuals experiencing serious symptoms [33].

The emphasis is on establishing some potential applications of intelligent speech processing for patients diagnosed with COVID-19. Analyzing voice recordings from these individuals can assist in developing audio-only-based models for intelligently categorizing patients' health states across four dimensions, including sickness severity, sleep quality, weariness, and anxiety. Two well-established acoustic feature sets and SVM are used for this purpose. The trials demonstrate that an average accuracy of 69% is reached when assessing disease severity according to treatment duration in days [34].

The criticality of the individual is predicted using an XGBoost ML method. The algorithm selects three critical clinical variables from over 300, including "lymphocyte, high-sensitivity C-reactive protein, and lactic dehydrogenase dyspnea". This three-index diagnostic prediction model can predict the risk of mortality, and present a therapeutic pathway for differentiating critical cases [35]. Another study investigated 21 clinical characteristics that differed significantly between severe and non-severe cases and utilized ML to develop a predictive model. 455 patients' data are amassed, and 11 discriminating variables are chosen for modeling in the training and validation sets [36].

Monitoring Symptoms

A novel framework is developed to identify COVID-19 utilizing the built-in sensors of smartphones. The concept is a low-cost solution, as most radiologists currently use smartphones for various daily tasks. Moreover, ordinary individuals could utilize the framework to detect viruses on their devices. Nowadays, smartphones are incredibly powerful due to the presence of fast processors, ample memory, and many sensors, such as cameras, microphones, temperature, inertial, proximity, color, humidity, and wireless chipsets. The framework powered by AI examines the signal data from the mobile device sensors to monitor the degree of seriousness of pneumonia and the outcome of the sickness [37]. Electronic health records of COVID-19 individuals are monitored through the integration of classical epidemiology methodologies, Natural Language Processing (NLP), and ML techniques, later utilized to forecast which patients should be admitted to the ICU [38].

COVID-19 EPIDEMIOLOGY

Predicting the disease's evolution is a significant challenge during the present pandemic. By developing a forecasting model, local authorities can improve their public health service's long-term planning, decreasing the fatality rate. Even though multiple traditional statistical modeling methodologies produce a reasonably accurate prediction of the pandemic, the complexities inherent in the data are frequently tricky to represent using traditional methods. An overview of different implementations of AI in COVID-19 Epidemiology is discussed in this portion of the chapter.

Pandemic Prediction

AI tools, especially ML and DL techniques, capture these time-sequence data complexities more effectively. As a result, numerous studies employ AI technologies to predict the pandemic better.

ML-based Forecasting

The purpose of this approach is to use supervised ML and "Empirical Bayesian Kriging (EBK)" methodologies to deduce the correlations and motifs of the epidemic in Sub-Saharan Africa (SSA). The estimate is based on cumulative time series data assembled by JHU on COVID-19 in SSA. COVID-19 observations are combined with sociodemographic and health marker survey results of SSA member nations that recorded identified infections and fatalities between March 1, 2020, and March 27, 2020. Lasso is used for selecting features and statistical deduction in the supervised ML process. Additionally, EBK is utilized to generate a raster, including information about the spatial dispensation of the COVID-19 epidemic [39].

Seven factors are shown to be considerably linked with the likelihood of COVID-19 illness using the lasso Cross-fit prediction model. According to this study, the germination period of SARS-CoV-2 is three days. The consistent three-day decline in the epidemic speed of change from 38% on April 24, 2020, to 24% on April 27, 2020, demonstrates the beneficial effect of nations' efforts to halt the pandemic. The extrapolated maps indicate that SARS-CoV-2 is increasing daily and seems to be localized to a small area in South Africa. In the provinces of West Africa, the new cases and mortality rate will probably increase [39].

According to certain studies, COVID-19 epidemic has seasonal transmission, incidence, and dispersion trends. In relation to the progress and dispersion of the virus, scientific analysis is needed to define whether the coming summer will be able to protect people from COVID-19. Numerous experts have been asked specifically whether extreme summer temperatures can curb the dissemination of COVID-19, as it happens with another seasonal ague. Given the numerous unsolved concerns and mysteries surrounding COVID-19, in-depth research and analysis of relevant weather phenomena are required. Additionally, comprehending the nature of COVID-19 and estimating its spread requires additional research on the actual influence of weather parameters on COVID-19 transmission among humans [40].

Several regressor ML models are proposed to determine the association between various parameters and the propagation rate of COVID-19. The ML techniques in this study analyses the influence of weather parameters, namely temperature and humidity, on COVID-19 propagation by identifying the link between reported cases and weather parameters in specific areas. To assess the suggested method, essential datasets on weather and census characteristics were gathered and underwent the appropriate preprocessing steps. The experimental findings indicate that weather parameters are more predictive of death than other census factors, namely population, age, and urbanism. As a result of this finding, it has been deduced that temperature and humidity are critical factors in forecasting COVID-19 death rates. Additionally, it is stated that as the temperature increases, the chances of contagion are reduced [40].

The effect of meteorological conditions, such as atmospheric conditions and contamination, on the dissemination of COVID-19, is analyzed. Additionally, communal and statistical indicators, namely Gross Domestic Product (GDP) per capita and population denseness, are also considered. By applying epidemiological theory, a paradigm for developing forecasting techniques to anticipate the transmission of COVID-19 is constructed. ML techniques, such as decision trees and different variants of SVM are utilized in the suggested framework. Given the nonlinear complexity of the observations, the radial kernel SVM, outperforms all other approaches and reports 96% of the variability. Consistent with the literature, this analysis reveals population density is the essential factor determining transmission. The univariate study demonstrates that increasing air pollution, population density and temperature contribute to spreading the disease. As an alternative, a rise in GDP can minimize the transmission [41].

A new SVM Regression approach is developed to investigate various SARS-CoV-2-related activities. The following are the five distinct tasks. (i) Forecasting COVID-19 transmission across locations. (ii) Comparing rates of growth and prevention strategies across nations. (iii) Predicting the course of the pandemic. (iv) Determining the virus's dissemination rate. (v) Finding a relation between COVID-19 and weather conditions. These task mentioned above benefits by unveiling information such as working and performance of mitigation techniques, patient recovery using former medications, progress, and end of the pandemic. Thus, support vectors are employed instead of simple regression lines to improve classification metrics. The technique is assessed and compared with other popular regression models on publicly available dataset. The favorable results manifest the model's excellence in both efficacy and veracity [42].

Clustering Strategies

A novel and timely way is proposed for accurately forecasting COVID-19 prevalence in China by combining illness predictions from rationalistic models with digital traces through explicable ML models. Significantly, the method is capable of producing reliable and precise forecasts two days in advance of the current time by incorporating (i) official health information from Chinese health authorities, (ii) COVID-19 relevant Baidu queries and responses (iii) media information broadcasted through Media Cloud (iv) day to day COVID-19 updates from a third-party mechanistic model called as GLEAM. The ML approach employs a clustering algorithm to exploit the geospatial synchronicity of COVID-19 prevalence throughout Chinese regions, and a data augmentation methodology to account for activities related to small outbreaks. The model transcends the benchmark models in 28 of China's 32 states, and it is recommended to additional countries and states presently afflicted by the COVID-19 pandemic to assist policymakers and authorities [43].

The COVID-19 pandemic has been identified as having its epicenter in New York City (NYC). An unsupervised ML methodology is proposed for identifying the inherent critical characteristics that are substantially connected with the growing rate of COVID-19 cases in NYC. On the conjecture that ZIP code regions with equivalent travel behavior, demography, and social economy will suffer similar epidemics, the most important parameters are selected for clustering and reduced to nine intelligible clusters. This clustering approach may assist the authorities in preventing the infection's transmission by using appropriate interventions [44].

A novel data-driven methodology for forecasting COVID-19 epidemic trends is presented. As a preparatory study, an LSTM network model is used. Even though this initial technique produced some unsatisfactory results, it provided an excellent benchmark for evaluating various ANN types. Following that, to determine important regions for validating ANN models. Clustering is performed using explicitly created features that describe a country's reaction to the pandemic's early transmission, and the resulting clusters are utilized to pick significant nations for training the models. These forecasts anticipate critical illness statistics, such as peak numbers and recorded cases. According to predictions, more than one million susceptible Brazilians may spread across the country's many provinces. The findings reveal that the epidemic is still spreading in Brazil, with transmission peaks expected after May 15 2020, in most areas. The end of COVID-19 pandemic will likely to occur between July and August 2020, depending on the region [45].

Neural Networks in Action

The purpose is to use official epidemiological information to anticipate the likely consequences of the COVID-19 outbreak using RNN powered by AI and then to analyze and evaluate the projected and observed data. The training dataset is created using publicly released datasets from the WHO and Johns Hopkins University (JHU) and then formed new prediction models using RNN with LSTM units. To compute the next predicted value, the data from the first 't' iterations are consolidated using a dense NN layer and a subsequent regression output layer. The comparison is made between expected, and observed values using root mean squared logarithmic errors (RMSLE), and then the estimated values are recalibrated [46].

The results suggest that the COVID-19 global epidemic is most likely a disseminated origin epidemic, and thus that repetitive spikes visualized using a graph are anticipated. The discrepancy between projected and verified information and proclivities is minimal. Policymakers, in particular, must be conscious that even if stringent public health practices are taken and maintained, further infectious maxima are feasible. AI-based forecasts may be practical tools for forecasting, and can update models in response to newly acquired data to gain a more accurate prediction of the contagion [46].

Due to the smaller number of daily samples available, data-driven approaches such as RNN may need to improve. To overcome this issue, an integrated spatiotemporal approach based on epidemic differential equations (ISEPE) and RNN is implemented. The previous is a compact method of a region's temporal contagion pattern after simplistic analysis and discretization, whereas the latter models the influence of nearby neighboring areas. The new model is capable of detecting hidden spatial information. The model is trained and evaluated upon pandemic observations collected in Italy, which surpasses available temporal models (SIR, dense NN and Auto-Regressive Integrated Moving Average (ARIMA)) in one-day three-day and 1-week advance forecasting, mainly when training data is scarce [47].

A novel forecasting strategy for COVID-19 instance prognosis is developed that utilizes GNN and movability datasets. In contradistinction to prevailing time series prediction approaches, the presented methodology comprehends from a "single large-scale spatio-temporal graph" where the nodes denote regional-wise people portability, edges indicate inter-regional interconnection based on human agility, and temporal denotes node features over a period. The technique is assessed on the US province COVID-19 observations, demonstrating that the GNN enriched spatial and temporal details enable the model to learn complicated behaviors. The results indicate a 6% decrease in RMSLE and an increase in absolute Pearson Correlation, equated to the moderately executing benchmark methods. When paired with GNN algorithms, this innovative source of knowledge can become a potential method for understanding the dissemination and progression of pandemic [48].

A primary objective for preventing subsequent accelerating transmission is to lower the disease contagion rate. The proposed algorithm utilizes AI in ascertaining causative factors associated with COVID-19 by examining previous repositories from "ourworldindata.org (Oxford University database)" and recently generated observations, as well as by assessing various univariate LSTM models for predicting instances and mortalities. As a result, it is shown that classical, layered, and bidirectional LSTM approaches dominate multilayer LSTM methods. Correlation analysis is also computed to assess the results, using many features such as population, exterior temperature, precipitation, sunshine, affected cases, Mortality, country, region, and population density from the previous three months, *i.e.*, January to March 2020 [49].

The cutting-edge DL techniques-oriented model is constructed to forecast COVID-19 outbreaks in Canada using JHU and the Canadian health authorities' datasets. This approach evaluates crucial elements to forecast the patterns and likely the end date of the present COVID-19 pandemic in Canada and throughout the globe. To estimate future COVID-19 instances, the LSTM network and DL technique are applied. According to the conclusion of the LSTM network, the pandemic might terminate as early as June 2020. Additionally, transmission rates among Canada, the United States of America, and Italy are evaluated by comparing. Forecasts in this approach are rendered using data accessed till March 30, 2020 [50].

Forecasting the extent of the COVID-19 epidemic on a regional and global scale is critical to implement essential promptitude plans and mitigation initiatives. Regional and global estimations are the result of the AI-based DL technique. This approach forecasts number of instances, the cumulative fatalities, and the everyday new instances. The cumulative instances are estimated for Europe and the Middle East, whereas everyday instances and the cumulative mortality rate are forecasted for China. The following ten days' values are forecasted using previously published factual COVID-19 time-series observations. For global estimates, Worldometers data is used. To estimate territorial and global forecasts, the DL architecture uses an LSTM layer, a dropout layer, and dense layers. The model is evaluated using the RMSE measure. Each day, the dissemination and circumstances change. This technique can adapt to this radical progress by retraining the DL model with new daily input and performing tangible predictions [51].

Forecasting Regression Models

Over the forthcoming days, a univariate time series technique is used to prognosticate COVID-19 instances in India. An ARIMA model is applied to observations obtained between January 30, 2020, and March 27, 2020, and it was validated using data amassed between March 28, 2020, and April 5, 2020. A nonlinear autoregressive (NAR) NN is built to examine models' efficiency. The algorithm forecasts COVID-19 cases every day for the upcoming 60 days. The study utilized statistical information from the "Ministry of Health and Family Welfare". The conclusion indicate a growing trajectory in actual and predicted COVID-19 instances, with roughly 1550 cases daily. The optimal ARIMA model was based on its "Bayesian Information Criteria (BIC)" scores, and resulted in a total R2 value of 0.96. The NAR model is composed of several neurons, and is enhanced using the "Levenberg-Marquardt optimization training algorithm" to achieve the maximum R2 value of 0.98 [52].

Iranian COVID-19 instances recorded between January 20, 2020, and February 29, 2020, were utilized to forecast the number of patients till April 30, 2020. Predictions were made using ANN and ARIMA models. The data was compiled using daily updates from the "Iran Ministry of Health" and free repositories made available by the JHU. To facilitate model evaluation, the observations are partitioned into a training and testing sets. The evaluation criterion is MSE and MAE. Both algorithms predicted that the number of newly infected individuals would grow exponentially. If the current transmission trend persists, daily infection numbers reported will be 7875 and 9560 by May 1, 2020, according to ARIMA and ANN. The model evaluation revealed that ARIMA perform better than ANN in forecasting the outcome [53].

The two primary issues are dealt with: (a) forecasting COVID-19 cases for different nations in the short term, and (b) risk estimation (in aspects of deaths) in a few tremendously infected nations by identifying multiple significant socio-demographic factors of the regions in addition to epidemic features. First issue is addressed by an intercrossed forecasting method based on ARIMA and Wavelet that can give twelve days in advance projections of the frequency of everyday affirmed instances in India, France, Canada, the United Kingdom, and South Korea. The prospective epidemic estimates for various countries will aid in the efficient deployment of medical facilities, ensure a quick caution mechanism for governing authorities. An optimum regression tree technique is used in the second challenge, to identify critical causative features that substantially impact mortality rates across many nations. This data-driven investigation will undoubtedly shed light on the study of rapid risk estimation in fifty severely impacted countries [54].

Polynomial regression and NN models are created to forecast the number of infected individuals from various nations over the time of fifteen days. Predictive analytics is performed on time series information transfigured on a logarithmic scale. Due to the confined number of training observations for every nation, an "Extreme Learning Machine (ELM)" is implemented to eliminate high variance. Since the time sequence observations are non-stationary, the sliding window method is utilized to obtain a correct forecast [55].

The short-duration COVID-19 projection model is proposed to forecast states and union territories of India, utilizing trending observations from February 29, 2020, to May 22, 2020. Ten-days estimates of the anticipated number of affected individuals and Mortality in India for April 23, 2020, to May 2, 2020, are derived using "Holt's second-order exponential smoothing method" and an ARIMA model. By May 2, 2020, the aggregate number of victims in India is expected to reach 36336, while the number of fatalities is expected to reach 1099. Additionally, the country is separated into serious regions according to the aggregate number of cases. Maharashtra is anticipated to be the most afflicted province, with a cumulative case count of about 9787 by May 2, 2020. On the other hand, Kerala and Karnataka are anticipated to move from the danger zone (*i.e.,* the most afflicted territory) to the less infected state. Gujarat and Madhya Pradesh, on the other side, will enter the danger zone. These findings indicate which states may be released from lockdown by May 3, 2020 [56].

Containment of the Pandemic

To control the epidemic, it is critical to maintain the rate of transmission low. Many AI-based methodologies are suggested and implemented to manage COVID-19 and reduce infection rates.

Evaluation of Risk

Determining the risk of transmission in each metropolitan area is critical for governments and authorities to develop policies for restoration. Standardization of an index for predicting the likelihood of spread in metropolitan regions to assist local governments in determining the most effective measures for reducing or restarting local activity under lockdown circumstances. The purpose is to develop a helpful tool for predicting the risk of transmission in urban regions by analyzing socioeconomic information such as the existence of events, enterprises, organizations, and the number of diseases [57].

The factorial formula-based suggested indicator is simple for specialists to apply. It is calibrated with the help of an optimization technique using datasets from 258 urban centers in the Apulian province (Italy). Additionally, a sophisticated analysis based on ANN training is executed to relate to phenomenon's nonlinearity. The assessment measures the effect of each factor on the likelihood of transmission, allowing for risk analysis and forecasting scenarios [57].

An increasing number of regions reporting native sectoral community spread would be a major setback in the fight against COVID-19. They highlight the imperative need for extensive monitoring to comprehend the transmission of COVID-19 and thus react with admissible society mitigation strategies. By extending the functionality of AI and maximizing massive and real-time observations obtained from heterogeneous sources, an AI-based approach (α-satellite) is implemented to detect and mitigate disease proactively. More precisely, given a specific destination (either *via* user intervention or automatic positional awareness), the established model will spontaneously deliver risk assessment information for that location in a hierarchical order *(e.g.,* nation, province, zone, place) to encourage people to choose good preventive actions while reducing interruptions to daily life [58].

Ensuring Safety Measures

People infected with SARS-CoV-2 are quarantined to prevent the virus from spreading. The medical science expert community has yet to devise a medicine to cure or improve the health condition of COVID-19 patients. The only way to guard against this virus is to follow the safety guidelines such as; maintaining a safe distance limit in the crowd, wearing masks and gloves, and frequently rinsing and sanitizing the hands. Government and policymaking authorities are engaged in prohibiting people from moving between cities to minimize transmission and monitor individuals in accordance with safety guidelines [59].

However, the authorities cannot monitor all the locations, including marketplaces, ATMs, banks, job premises, clinics, and hospitals and encourage individuals to observe safety recommendations. The purpose is to establish a novel approach to protect people from infected individuals and symptomatic (cough or fever) people. To validate the suggested technique, various CNN models are developed. The proposed AI-based monitoring system can be used with other tools to proactively monitor people adhering to safety requirements in various locations. With these preventative measures in place, humanity can overcome COVID-19 [59].

Social distancing is an approved efficacious method for controlling the transmission of COVID-19. On the other hand, people are not accustomed to maintaining a 2-meter (6-foot) separation among themselves. Dynamic surveillance systems competent in identifying and notifying persons about gaps between them can help prevent the epidemic's progression. Additionally, assessing social density in a selected area and controlling inflow might reduce the likelihood of social distancing infringement. On the contrary, collecting data and naming those who breach the regulations will abuse the rights of an individual in liberal societies [60].

An AI-based instantaneous social distancing sensing and alert system that takes into account four essential ethical considerations: (1) the application must be user -friendly, (2) human superintendent must be avoided in the tracking functionality, (3) cautions must not be directed at a specific person and (4) the application is configured to save no data. Concerning this context, a system is proposed to assess the social distance using a monocular camera and DL-based live entity detectors. If an infringement is spotted, a courteous caution signal is delivered to the person rather than identifying and criticizing social distancing guidelines' violators. Additionally, if the societal compactness exceeds a predetermined threshold, the device transmits a control signal to stabilize people's inflow rate. The suggested method is evaluated on real-world observations. The solution is deployable, and scripts are open-sourced [60].

Inspired by social distancing, a DL framework is proposed to automate the activity of inspecting social distance with the help of observation footage. The application uses the YOLO version-3 object recognition algorithm to distinguish persons from environmental noise and the Deepsort technique to trace detected individuals using bordering boxes and issued IDs. The YOLO v3 model's outcomes are compared with famous cutting-edge models. Subsequently, the paired vector representation L2 norm is calculated using the centered coordinates and bordering box dimensions to create a 3D feature space. The infringement indicator value is suggested to measure the violation of societal separation etiquette. The observational study revealed that the YOLO v3 integrated Deepsort trailing strategy delivered satisfying results [61].

SIRNet, a new hybrid ML model that integrates epidemiological models, is presented for anticipating the transmission of the COVID-19 pandemic. Along with community-weighted intensity and other nearby observations, characterized spatiotemporally detailed cellular mobility data is utilized as a substitute indicator for physical separation. At various geographical scales, it is proved that the range of physical separation choices currently under consideration by policymakers has epidemiologically significant repercussions spanning from viral extermination to proximate-total population predominance. The present intonation points in mobility differ per geographical location. SIRNet experiments offer primary constraints on this type of localized mobility that asymptotically induces confinement. The model can investigate non-pharmacological therapies, ways to decrease societal causalities, and long-term control mechanisms [62].

Due to the pandemic crisis, all economic activity and, consequently, production at industrial units across the majority of industries was halted. While it is critical to recommence manufacturing, it is even more critical to guarantee the safety of the plant's personnel. According to reports, avoiding social contact and wearing face masks while at work significantly minimizes the chance of infection. On CCTV feeds, computer vision technology is used to monitor employee activities and detect infringements that generate real-time speech alarms in the workplace. A cost-effective and economical technique is described for utilizing AI to establish a safe workplace in a factory environment. The concept is demonstrated by developing a robust algorithm for measuring social separation using a combination of state-of-the-art DL and conventional projective geometry methods. The approach is being implemented across the Aditya Birla Group's production units. It has been observed that the face mask identification system has a high degree of accuracy when used with various customized masks [63].

Wearing a proper facemask is essential for infection prevention and control; their efficiency has been compromised, primarily due to incorrect wearing. By integrating ultra-resolution photos and classification networks, a new approach is developed for identifying face mask-wearing conditions. The system addresses a tri-class classification challenge based on 2D facial photos. The intended approach is divided into four stages: photo preprocessing, facial recognition and clipping, photo ultra-resolution and detection of facemask-wearing situations. The technique is trained and assessed on the publicly available Clinical Masks Dataset, which contains 3838 photos, with 672 photos of individuals not wearing a facemask, 135 photos of individuals wearing a facemask incorrectly, and 3031 photographs of individuals wearing a facemask correctly. Finally, the suggested DL model obtained an accuracy of 99% and surpassed existing facemask detecting approaches. The results demonstrate that this model can identify facemask-wearing situations efficiently, suggesting that it could be used to mitigate COVID-19 outbreaks [64].

Combating False Information

Social media is critical during epidemic diseases such as COVID-19 because it allows individuals to instantly communicate news, personal observations and perspectives to a global audience. A model is created after examining how the motivating factors, personal characteristics, and broadcasting of doubtful information during COVID-19 persuaded social media. The model utilizes the data amassed from youngsters in Bangladesh and works based on structural equation modeling and NN approaches. The outcomes indicate that the individuals motivated by self-promotion and amusement, and those with impaired self-regulation, are more inclined to distribute dubious information. Exploration and spirituality were found to be negatively associated with the dissemination of dubious information [65].

On the internet, a flood of possibly precarious COVID-19 falsehoods is circulating. The content of COVID-19 is quantified using ML among internet critics of established health advice, particularly vaccinations ("anti-vax"). The anti-vax society is shown to be less engaged in COVID-19 than the pro-vaccination ("pro-vax") society. The anti-vax society, on the contrary, has a wider spectrum of "varieties" of COVID-19 themes and thus attracts more people attempting COVID-19 advice online. As a result, the anti-vax group appears to be more assertive to gain new support in the future than the pro-vax group. This is problematic because if a COVID-19 vaccine is not widely adopted, the world will miss the mark of ensuring multitude immunity, leaving nations vulnerable to future COVID-19 renaissances. A mechanistic model is designed to evaluate these observations and to aid in determining the potential success of intervention options. The adaptable, approach addresses the high-priority issue of social media platforms analyzing massive amounts of online health misconceptions and deception [66].

The eruption of falsehoods coming along with the COVID-19 outbreak has overwhelmed fact-reviewers and news organizations globally, posing a new big challenge for government responses. Not only does misinformation foster ambiguity about the medical field among civilians, but it also magnifies skepticism in government officials and legislative bodies. To assist in addressing this issue, an AI-based approach for categorizing COVID-19 misinformation is devised. The COVID-19 misinformation categories are certainly used to: (i) direct fact-checking initiatives towards the most harmful types of COVID-19 misinformation; and (ii) guide authorities in their attempts to provide reliable public health statements and combat COVID-19 falsehoods. This approach also presents a corpus comprising the enormous collection of manually labeled COVID-19 misinformation categories and a classification-conscious neural model for COVID-19 misinformation categorization and topic exploration. It also facilitates an in-depth assessment of COVID-19 misinformation categories in terms of time, quantity, falsified form, content type, and source [67].

Rumors and conspiracy theories flourish in the circumstances fueled by uncertainty and distrust. As a result, it is unsurprising that one's on the pandemic are sprouting, provided the absence of any definitive meticulous research agreement on the pathogen, its propagation, control, or the pandemic's protracted societal and financial consequences. Among the storylines spreading like wildfire are those claiming that the: (i) COVID-19 is a myth propagated by an international clique, (ii) The pathogen (SARS-CoV-2) gets activated through 5G technology, (iii) the Chinese government is intentionally discharging the disease-causing virus as a bio-weapon into various societies and (iv) Bill Gates is trying to establish a universal vigilance administration by utilizing this virus as a tool. At the same time, few might disregard these narratives as having a negligible effect on real-world conduct. Contemporary occurrences such as property ruination, racially charged violence targeting Asian Americans, and demonstrations advocating for defiance of public health rules throw this conclusion into question [68].

Motivated by narration, social media websites and media reports are crawled to find the foundational storytelling frameworks that underpin these tales' development through ML approaches. It is illustrated how the diverse storytelling platforms that drive gossip, unauthentic information, illegitimate facts, and conspiracy theories depend on the convergence of apparently miscellaneous categories of information and how they relate to more extensive reporting on the pandemic. Tracking such affiliations, links and connections simultaneous could be valuable for detecting regions of content that are especially susceptible to misinterpretation by conspiracists. Understanding the characteristics of social networking narratives and the storytelling frameworks that generate these tales may also aid in developing techniques to stop their dissemination [68].

Managing the Consequences

The COVID-19 epidemic has profoundly affected numerous facets of human existence, commerce, and manufacturering. In certain studies, AI is employed to develop methods for mitigating the pandemic's impacts.

Energy Services

The COVID-19 pandemic has caused tremendous challenges for enterprises and grid operators worldwide. Globally, due to strong social distance regulations, power usage characteristics have evolved in size and everyday routines. These changes have created major difficulty in estimating short-term load. Although algorithms often incorporate weather, scheduling data, and historical intake levels as input factors, they cannot capture massive and abrupt shifts in socioeconomic behavior throughout a pandemic. To supplement the existing foundations of forecasting techniques, mobility is introduced as a metric of economic activity [69].

Mobility data provide accurate representations of population-level activities during the deployment and consequent relaxation of social distancing policies. The primary limitation of this dataset is that just a few instances with confined mobility are related to the current outbreak. To address this issue with less data, a TL technique is developed that facilitates knowledge transmission across many geographical locations. This architecture takes advantage of the diversity between these locations, and the resultant consolidated model can significantly improve the algorithm's performance in each region's day-ahead forecast. The suggested approach outperforms standard forecasting models by more than thrice in experiments for territories in the United States and Europe. Additionally, the suggested model is capable of projecting how power demand would recuperate under various mobility circumstances [69].

Considering the medical and technological advances over the last century, biological challenges such as the COVID-19 pandemic continue to threaten humanity. While one component of an epidemic is the loss of life, the epidemic has a wide range of consequences for local and international communities. A regressive, and NN model is created to study the influence of the pandemic on power and petrol fuel consumption in China. The ecological analysis demonstrates that the outbreak's severity considerably impacts energy and petroleum demand, both internally and externally. According to the model's results, the resilience of petrol fuel and power necessity for the infected patients is -0.15% and -0.66%, respectively. The findings demonstrate that outbreak status considerably effects on power demand and also has ramifications throughout the human community [70].

Assisting the Organizations

Among the numerous challenges raised by the current COVID-19 pandemic is charities' ability to react to disasters and uphold their trustee and moral obligations to use funds efficiently and for the desired causes. A technological solution is proposed to tackle the issues faced by charitable organizations in China and other places. The existing predicament must be regarded as a rallying cry for the technology sector, which possesses the necessary needs, regulations, and infrastructure to dramatically alter the entire perspective of pandemic reaction and charity governance by deploying of AI tools. Fundamental adjustments are required in the framework and methodology to deal with such emergencies. The moment has come for worldwide technologists to collaborate on developing transnational solutions to pressing humanitarian catastrophes [71].

AI has generated great excitement and has transitioned to revitalize nearly every field, including the legal profession. New legal simulated AI application such as Ross intelligence, combined with ML and NLP, provides workable fight objectives, increased legal clarity, and increased access to justice, as well as new challenges to traditional law corporations that provide legal services utilizing an influenced cohort correlate model. Additionally, lawyer bots powered by AI are undertaking duties that would ordinarily need human intelligence. A query emerges in such a scenario: can these AI-built lawyer bots eventually supplant intelligent human attorneys? As the world is confronted with the problems inflicted by the worldwide pandemic, this subject becomes even more critical [72].

How COVID-19 situation will alter the justice delivery system, and what is its resemblance? An approach is proposed to assess the importance of AI in altering the justice delivery system in the aftermath of COVID-19. The study seeks to explore the many ways in which AI influences the legal profession, determine how it impacts legal employment, evaluate the duties in the legal field that AI cannot perform, and discuss the legal concerns surrounding its AI implementation. Additionally, the report makes recommendations for the legal industry's future, assisting professionals and scholars [72].

Online purchases are growing in popularity, particularly in the life-threatening situation of the COVID-19 pandemic. Governments have now urged citizens to do as many transactions as possible without using cash. Practically speaking, it is often challenging to incorporate it into every transaction. Due to the rapid increase in the frequency of such cashless payments during the COVID-19 shutdown timeframe, fraudulent transactions are escalating significantly. Cheating can be detected by examining a customer's previous transaction history. Typically, banks or other transactions administrators notify consumers about a transaction if they discover any divergence from established norms. Banks and credit card lenders are using various technologies to identify fraud during COVID-19, including decision trees, rule-based mining, ML, NN, data mining, and fuzzy grouping. These strategies attempt to ascertain a customer's conventional pattern based on their previous behaviors [73].

The purpose of a new approach is to excavate fraudulent transactions that occur in such an insurmountable position. Cybercriminals frequently target digital payment systems. Detecting fraudulent transactions during money transfers may help protect clients from monetary loss. A novel framework is proposed for monitoring and detecting fraudulent behavior using DL. Deceitful interactions are recognized by utilizing RNN to a simulated financial dataset created by PaySim. The proposed technique of detecting misleading transactions shows an F1-Score of 99% [73].

Education and Sports

The outbreak of COVID-19 in several nations has resulted in a shift from conventional face-to-face lecturing to online learning systems, which directly impacts educational quality. Using user contentment on Chinese educational software platforms as a research focus, a web spider or robot and a set of questionnaires in form of survey are used to gather information on online and offline user experiences, a client gratification indicator scheme is constructed using emotion analysis and available literature for statistical analysis, and a backpropagation NN model is developed to predict user contentment. The finding demonstrates that the consumers' characteristics exhibit an indirect effect on client contentment, whereas system accessibility depicts the largest impact. Finally, recommendations are made to enhance the online education system to raise the rate of online learning during a pandemic [74].

Almost all main league sports are canceled or delayed indefinitely in the aftermath of COVID-19. The sports sector has taken a significant hit due to the incertitude surrounding future sporting events. Numerous situations have been explored regarding how and when sporting could resume. The proposed work explores several possibilities about the impact of supporters' presence or lacking, on important League Baseball squad performance in the circumstances of physical separation and other COVID-19 safety guidelines. The approach replicates the win-loss probabilities for multiple situations and assesses each squad's local influence using information from the 2017-2019 tournaments [75].

The model illustrates that a specific team's domestic influence is proportional between domicile and outside and that players are unlikely to win or lose extra matches in unbiased sports venues, like players getting a strong domicile ground influence will lose enough square sports, obliged to play at domicile still have the chance of winning more fair and balanced games that might be played in the distant venue. on the other hand, single sports will have a distinct outcome due to the imbalance of the domicile effect between sides. The simulation indicates that these minor alterations in individual games can result in a small variation in contest positions between a full spell, a half spell, and a full spell with no supporters. This evaluation assists decision-makers in determining the impact of the changing circumstances on individual squad performance as they train for the 2020 tournament spells [75].

PHARMACEUTIC APPLICATIONS

Discovering an effective medication can contribute to lowering the disease's fatality rate. Three primary therapeutic possibilities for the condition are drug repurposing or repositioning, investigational remedies such as remedesivir, and immunotherapies (vaccine). Repurposing medications with low adverse effects for disease therapy is a critical and optimistic technique for generating novel therapeutic options. In certain studies, AI technologies are employed to combat COVID-19. As the epidemic progresses, AI technologies have the capabilities, recommended to be used in drug evaluation and repositioning phases.

Drug Repositioning

The examination of pharmaceuticals currently on the market and being used to treat different diseases in order to expedite patient recovery, in other words, repurposing or repositioning already available drugs. COVID-19 treatment strategies included repurposing existing drugs, developing new medicines such as redeliver, and developing a vaccination. Among these initiatives, combination therapy based on pharmacological repositioning is one of the most actively pursued. Historically, multi-drug therapies have been constructed by choosing medications depending on their operation mechanism. This is accompanied by dose optimization to maximize drug collaboration. This strategy is frequently utilized in the creation and repositioning of drugs. On the other hand, fulfilling synergistic associations is a significantly distinct conclusion from universally optimizing association therapy, which aims to achieve the greatest feasible therapeutic outcome using a mixture of candidate medicines and dosages for a given illness indication [76].

The outcomes of Project IDentif.AI are presented to tackle this difficulty. Within four days of project commencement, an AI-oriented system is utilized to query a huge 13-drug/dose parameter span, fast generating responsive association treatment that efficiently reduces animal virus contagion of A549 lung cells.

Notably, a sevenfold variation in efficiency is shown when the highest combination is dosed optimally versus sub-optimally, highlighting the vital necessity of identifying the optimal drug and dose mixture. The framework is illness portent and mechanism-skeptic and used to build extremely effective and tolerated therapeutic regimens on an N-of-1 and inhabitant scale. Additionally, this approach analyzes critical issues from medical economics to international healthcare policy that may contribute to the platform's widespread deployment to combat COVID-19 and future epidemics [76].

The enormous complexity of medication design and clinical trial methods frequently precludes the rapid development of novel therapeutic formulations for this pandemic. Recent advances in computer power and ML techniques have been used to alter the drug development procedure. As a result, a comprehensive study of ML for medicinal agent repositioning is needed. An ML model is proposed based on the NB method that marks a metric of approximately Ă=74% in predicting the medications, utilized to treat COVID-19. The study suggests that approximately ten FDA-sanctioned commercial medications could be repurposed. The three medications meet the criteria well, with the antiviral drug Amprenavir (DrugBank ID–DB00701) having the maximum efficacy based on the chosen standards. The proposed work can assist medical professionals in being more precise in their search for and testing COVID-19 therapy molecules. As described here, the ML-based method of drug discovery can be a prospective intelligent drug design technique for communal purposes [77].

The COVID-19 outset underscores the significance of rapidly, certain and reliably prioritizing clinically licensed medicines for their potential efficacy against SARS-CoV-2) contagion. AI, network proximity and diffusion-based algorithms are used to rate 6,345 medicines based on their predicted efficiency towards SARS-CoV-2. To validate the forecasts, 920 medications are used, that were systematically examined in VeroE6 cells, and a collection of pharmaceuticals now undergoing medical testing that reflects the clinical community's evaluation of prospective COVID-19 efficiency. It is explored that no specific predictive algorithm can consistently producing credible results on all COVID-19 data repositories and parameters. This observation inspired to build of a multimodal approach capable of fusing the estimates of many methods since it was discovered that an agreement between the various predictive approaches routinely outperforms the efficiency of the best specific pipelines [78].

The top-rated medicines are examined in human cells and obtained a 63% success rate, compared to a 0.8% success rate in unguided tests. Four of the six medications that decreased viral illness could be potentially repurposed to combat COVID-19, implying the possibility of novel COVID-19 therapies. Additionally, it is discovered that 77 of the 78 medicines that helped minimize viral contagion did not bind the SARS-CoV-2-targeted proteins, suggesting that these network medications operate *via* network-oriented processes that cannot be detected using docking-oriented methodologies. These advancements paved the way for indentifying repurposable medications for future infections and ignored illnesses that are overlooked by the high prices and lengthy timetable associated with new drug development [78].

Currently, there shortage efficient COVID-19 medicines. The potential for developing COVID-19 preventive and therapeutic techniques through drug repositioning is quite encouraging. An extensive knowledge graph is constructed from a massive scientific corpus of approximately 24 million PubMed articles, comprising 15 million links covering 39 interactions linking medications, illnesses, proteins/genes, routes, and transcription. "41 repurposable drugs (including dexamethasone, indomethacin, niclosamide, and toremifene)" are identified whose medicinal correlations with COVID-19 are corroborated using RNA transcripts and protein expression data from SARS-CoV-2 contaminated living cells and information from progressive medical investigations, using Amazon computational cloud service and a DL framework. The proposed methodology does not recommend any specific medicine; it provides a robust DL methodology for prioritizing current pharmaceuticals for further exploration, which can speed up COVID-19 medication development [79].

Immune System Analysis

There is a compelling need to develop therapeutic targets and medications that will allow COVID-19 victims to be adequately treated. In silico investigations of the body's immune protein molecular interaction structure, unit-cell RNA sequencing of living tissue, and ANN are used to identify possible therapeutic targets for COVID-19 medication repositioning. 27 prospective therapeutic targets are found in goblet cells, type II alveolar cells and intestinal absorptive cells of patients with various immunopathologies after screening 1,585 tight-confidence immune system proteins. A fully connected DNN is used to pick the ideal multiclass classification model for predicting the function of 10,673 drugs, resulting in multiple authorized drugs, substances under examination, and exploratory compounds with the best AUC. These medications can be suggested for the treatment of acute COVID-19 individuals after they have been thoroughly evaluated in clinical trials [80].

Thousands of people are killed by rapid and undetectable virus mutations before the immune response can generate a suppressive antibody. Tens of thousands will be saved if fast approaches for identifying peptides or antibody structures are developed to suppress the viral antigenic determinant of SARS-CoV-2. A distinct ML approach is proposed to predict potential suppressive synthetic immunoglobulins for SARS-CoV-2. 1934 virus-antibody sequences are gathered along with corresponding clinical patient neutralizing responses to train an ML model to forecast antibody reaction. Applying the graph feature technique and multiple ML models, several speculative antibody sequences are examined; as a result, nine consistent antibodies are found that possibly curb SARS-CoV-2. Many fields of science like computational biology, molecular structure analysis and molecular movement-based computer simulations are integrated to examine the permanence of the person's antibodies that prevent SARS-CoV-2 [81].

Exploring the Molecular Structure of Medicine

An AI technique is suggested to analyze resemblance based on infinitesimal structure and the situation in which operational clusters are grouped by 3D dispersion of pharmacophores to locate descendant medicines comparable to the ancestor that were formerly evaluated for the pandemic. ML methods are utilized to assess a set of 78 antiviral compounds and their constitutional information to uncover viable emergency therapies. A DL Algorithm is utilized to find chemical structures that may be possible viral antagonists. An *in vitro* pharmacological therapy is undertaken to demonstrate its efficacy. Dependable molecular connection data is provided as a foundation for therapeutic protein-protein communication structures, which serve as essential data repositories. These networks are analyzed using a DL technique. The program can identify obscure linkages between medications and human proteins that the pathogen seeks to bind [82–86].

Vaccine Development

ML algorithms are employed in the production of vaccines. To anticipate vaccine individuals, the Vaxign reversal vaccinology technique and the recently created "Vaxign-ML" ML technology are employed. AI algorithms are utilized to research virus mutation characteristics in order to produce vaccines. It is proposed that "bacille Calmette-Guerin vaccination (a tuberculosis vaccine)" can decrease COVID-19's intensity [87–89].

UNDERSTANDING THE CONTAGION PATHOGEN

Understanding the contagion pathogen (SARS-CoV-2) and its characteristics is a major difficulty in pandemic management. In this field, some study employs AI technologies. The bioinformatics of this virus, which corresponds with the human population, must be understood as soon as possible. The categorization of COVID-19 Human Protein Sequences (HPS) by nation is proposed using ML algorithms. The proposed model classifies 9239 sequences through three phases: data preprocessing, data tagging, and evaluation. The data preprocessing tool transforms the amino acids of SARS-CoV-2 HPS into nine sets of numerals on the basis of magnitude and polarity. It employs the "conjoint triad" technique. There are two ways for classifying data representing 27 nations ranging from 0 to 26 in phase two [90].

The first technique assigns one value to each nation based on their tag numerals, while the second is based on binary values for every nation. ML techniques are employed in the last phase to find diverse COVID-19 HPS according to their nations. Using a linear SVM classifier, the nation-based binary tagging approach yielded Ă=100%, Ŝ=100%, and Ş=90%. Furthermore, because the United States has a large amount of disease information, it is more likely to be classified correctly than other nations with less information. The uneven information for COVID-19 HPS is a critical challenge, particularly given that the access data from the United States account for 76% of overall 9239 sequences. The proposed model can be utilized to predict COVID-19 HPS in various nations [90].

Major viral infestations necessitate an early explanation of taxonomy and the genesis of the viral genomic sequences (GS) for the planning process, confinement, and therapeutics. A study reveals an innate SARS-CoV-2 genomic signature and combines it with an ML-based alignment-free technique to quickly, robustly, and precisely categorize of the entire SARS-CoV-2 GS. The suggested approach incorporates digital signal processing and supervised ML to perform GS analysis, reinforced by a DT model. A Spearman's rank correlation coefficient is used for output verification. These techniques are implemented to evaluate a substantial data repository of above 6000 distinct viral GS comprising 62 million bp, along with 30 SARS-CoV-2 GS accessible on January 30, 2020 [91].

The findings confirm the concept of bat ancestry and categorize the SARS-CoV-2 as a Sarbecovirus within the Betacoronavirus family. The model achieves a classification Ă=100% and explores the most pertinent associations between (5000) viral GS in no time, using only raw DNA sequence records and no specific biomedical expertise, mentoring and GS mappings. This shows that for new viruses and pathogenic GS, the alignment-free whole-genome ML technique can give a viable, realistic choice for Phylogenetic classification [91].

The SARS-CoV-2 RNA pathogen is capable of causing mutations in the living human cell. Accurately determining gene modification rates is critical for understanding the development of the pathogen and determining the threat of emerging active infection. A study investigates the changes in the entire GS derived from infected individuals' datasets from various nations. The obtained dataset is analyzed to detect nucleotide alteration and codon alterations independently. Additionally, the observed mutation rate is classified for four separate areas (United States, Australia, China and remaining countries) depending on the size of the dataset [92].

In comparison to other nucleotides, a large proportion of Adenine (A) and Thymine (T) is found to be altered. However, codons do not mutate as frequently as nucleotides. SARS-CoV-2 pathogen's eventual mutation rate has been predicted using an RNN-based LSTM model. The LSTM method achieves an optimized RMSE of 0.059 in the validation phase and 0.039 in the training phase. Applying this approach, the GS modification pace of the 500th individual at a future time is estimated. It is realized that if more clinical information is available in continuous time, this methodology is designed to estimate daily genetic changes [92].

Several techniques are being investigated, including protease and Glycosylated Spike Protein (GSP) inhibitors, which delineate the major fusion point between SARS-CoV-2 and pathogen invaded cells. Regardless, the "Heptad Repeat 1 (HR1)" motif on the GSP is the least mutable locus and thus the most promising candidate for novel inhibitor medicines. The suggested method differs from others because it involves the proper training of a DNN against SARS-CoV-2. A Siamese Neural Network (SNN) is implemented to distinguish the entire virus protein code from HIV-1 and Ebola [93].

The current DL model perfectly understands the peptide connection of the SARS-CoV-2 protein structure. Unlike previous efforts, it is not relatively easily trained on publicly available datasets with no ligand-peptide knowledge of SARS-CoV-2. Remarkably, the SNN exhibits a $\hat{S}$ = 84% for peptide affinity categorization, with 3028 peptides from the SATPdb library demonstrating a $\S$ = 94% for the peptide. Because multiple scientific articles have previously depicted immune inhibitory medication, a major suppressor of peptide inhibits the replication of many pathogens, including SARS-CoV-2 and MERS-CoV, this synergy between peptide and HR1 can offer new possibilities for exploration [93].

According to various comparative studies using the virus GS, bats or pangolins may have been the virus's ancestral carriers. The origin of the SARS-CoV-2 is investigated using AI and raw virus GS. Unsupervised clustering algorithms examine and evaluate more than 300 GS of COVID-19 victims gathered from several nations. The results of several AI- empowered tests utilizing clustering algorithms show that all SARS-CoV2 GS investigated correspond to a group including bat and pangolin coronavirus GS. This lends substantial credence to scientific claims that bats and pangolins are likely carriers for SARS-CoV-2.

Considering GS analysis, the research suggests that bats are more inclined than pangolins to be SARS-CoV-2 pathogen hosts [94].

CONCLUSION

There is only appropriate medication against COVID-19 on the current date (October 5, 2021). Because of the swift surge in the number of patients and the massive financial consequences it has caused, there is a necessity for viable pharmaceutical measures. Rapid identification, prediction, and medication of COVID-19 instances are critical in mitigating harm. Governments worldwide are making extreme efforts, with massive financial impacts, to mitigate the effects of the outbreak. Strategies based on AI offer viable solutions to many of today's problems. This chapter addresses the use of AI in combatting and managing the effects of COVID-19. To date, AI techniques have produced largely satisfying outcomes. Even though many AI applications are explored in the context of COVID-19 studies, many areas still need AI implementations to solve the present issue. This section addresses the issues these systems confront and offers solutions for dealing with them.

• AI applications require a lot of input data to get reliable outcomes; hence it is a disadvantage as such with AI systems. It is especially true for techniques like DL, which are prone to overfitting. The first step should be for the community to create a single forum for scholars to share data. Specifying data gathering norms such as file formats, type of information gathered, tagging, and codes is also critical. It is especially problematic in hospitals because data is difficult to disseminate.

• Because different institutions and authorities have distinct data gathering processes, the type and structure of previously gathered data can change greatly. Data fusion techniques should be used to create a single dataset. Evaluating other data fusion approaches for the problem is recommended as a topic of future research.

• The RT-PCR method is typically utilized for COVID-19 screening, which could be more precise. Lack of smell, indications such as body discomfort, fever, and clinical test information as discussed above, can be symptomatic of the condition. For more exact results, the creation of ensemble models is recommended to take any form of discriminative information from diverse tests as input.

• Many studies have shown that analyzing vocal signals can be useful in collecting vital data about individuals. To the best of my knowledge, there hasn't been any research into using vocal sounds to detect SARS-CoV-2 infected individuals. Coughing is a key sign of the condition and coughing in influenza or other illnesses is much more different than the coughing in COVID-19 victims. Analyzing cough vocal impulses for diagnosing and estimating a patient's seriousness can be viewed as future work.

• Most epidemiological studies consider only a subset of the productive characteristics or parameters in the analysis. For example, they are just considering parameters like weather, government regulation, and so on. Numerous factors can influence the contagion. A thorough investigation of the factors influencing the replication rate should be carried out. These parameters should then be evaluated for analysis and prediction in any epidemiology study.

• Many ML challenges are optimization concerns. More specifically, it is an optimization challenge to train a multilayer NN. Since gradient descent algorithms are a core part of prevailing and conventional techniques, they are susceptible to being stuck in localized optima. Hence in the future, while tackling COVID-19 relevant tasks, global search techniques should be used to train these models.

• The pandemic has increased xenophobia and hatred of persons of different ethnicity. It is unquestionably a menace to human rights that must be addressed as soon as possible. Learning the mechanics of this occurrence is another difficulty that AI techniques can handle.

• Fitness trackers, and mobile sensors, including smart watches, are frequently used. These can be a foundation for creating AI systems for diagnostics, observation, and consulting purposes. These gadgets are meant to collect data for symptoms such as temperature, oxygen saturation, coughs, and so on, as well as people's travel history, and store it in a central registry. The repository can then be utilized to train AI models for diagnostics or healthcare advice. The information can also be utilized for clinical purposes, such as delivering appropriate caution to individuals and officials to implement remedies such as sterilization, social distancing, and quarantine procedures.

• All of the methodologies discussed in this chapter involve abstract AI techniques, and to the extent literature survey, there has yet to be remarkable progress in developing easily interpretable AI solutions. An explicable AI approach is when the developed application is made to deliver knowledge and intuition into how the designed model arrived at the outcome. It is especially essential in diagnostics, where AI systems aid physicians. As the technology would act as an advisor in this scenario, the rationale that the AI algorithms suggest a specific solution or prognosis should be performed is critical in educating the ultimate decision-maker.

• This COVID-19 outbreak will end one day, but its long-term effects on the economy, public health, academia, commerce, international relationships, *etc.*, will be felt. It is critical to understand how the disease's complexities will manifest in the upcoming days so that the solutions can be deduced at the initial stage because it is often easier to control in their inception. Only now, there has been a lot of study done in anticipating these domains. AI techniques can be used to forecast and provide solutions to challenges that humankind may confront in the future.

• One significant problem is bridging the gap between research and effect. There is a lot of study and innovation regarding establishing new AI systems, but seeing them implemented in reality is another story. More close collaboration between researchers and practitioners is required.

Although numerous fascinating use cases implement AI to solve the complexities caused by the epidemic, as listed above, many sectors are still to be explored and managed. This SARS-CoV-2 outbreak has given a formidable task for AI to demonstrate its use in extraordinary factual challenges. If AI is proficient in tackling significant issues, then extra societal acceptance is assured.

ACKNOWLEDGEMENTS

All authors contributed to the study's conception and design. Material preparation, data collection and analysis were performed by Mohamed Yousuff and Rajasekhara Babu. Anusha and Matheen wrote the first draft of the manuscript and all authors commented on previous versions of the manuscript. All authors read and approved the final manuscript.

REFERENCES

[1]   M. Cascella, M. Rajnik, A. Aleem, S.C. Dulebohn, and R. Di Napoli, Features, Evaluation, and Treatment of Coronavirus (COVID-19).*StatPearls (Internet)* StatPearls Publishing: Treasure Island, FL, 2021.

[2]   "WHO Coronavirus (COVID-19) Dashboard World Health Organization", Available at: https://covid19.who.int/(Accessed on: Sep. 10, 2021).

[3]   M.S. Razai, K. Doerholt, S. Ladhani, and P. Oakeshott, "Coronavirus disease 2019 (COVID-19): a guide for uk gps", *B.M.J,* vol. 368, p. m800, 2020.
[http://dx.doi.org/10.1136/bmj.m800] [PMID: 32144127]

[4]   L. Browning, R. Colling, E. Rakha, N. Rajpoot, J. Rittscher, J.A. James, M. Salto-Tellez, D.R.J. Snead, and C. Verrill, "Digital pathology and artificial intelligence will be key to supporting clinical and academic cellular pathology through COVID-19 and future crises: the pathlake consortium perspective", *J. Clin. Pathol.,* vol. 74, no. 7, pp. 443-447, 2021.
[http://dx.doi.org/10.1136/jclinpath-2020-206854] [PMID: 32620678]

[5]   M.H. Tayarani N, "Applications of artificial intelligence in battling against COVID-19: a literature review", *Chaos Solitons Fractals,* vol. 142, p. 110338, 2021.
[http://dx.doi.org/10.1016/j.chaos.2020.110338] [PMID: 33041533]

[6]   *Machine Learning Yearning.,* 2018.

[7]   I. Goodfellow, Y. Bengio, and A. Courville, *Deep Learning.* MIT Press, 2016.

[8]   X. Pu, K. Chen, J. Liu, J. Wen, S. Zhneng, and H. Li, "Machine learning-based method for interpreting the guidelines of the diagnosis and treatment of COVID-19", *Sheng Wu I Hsueh Kung Cheng Hsueh Tsa Chih,* vol. 37, no. 3, pp. 365-372, 2020.
       [PMID: 32597076]

[9]   H. Obinata, "Can artificial intelligence predict the need for oxygen therapy in early stage COVID-19 pneumonia?", In: *Res. Sq.,* 2021.

[10]   A.S. Albahri, J.R. Al-Obaidi, A.A. Zaidan, O.S. Albahri, R.A. Hamid, B.B. Zaidan, A.H. Alamoodi, and M. Hashim, "Multi-biological laboratory examination framework for the prioritization of patients with COVID-19 based on integrated ahp and group vikor methods", *Int. J. Inf. Technol. Decis. Mak,* vol. 19, no. 5, pp. 1247-1269, 2020.
       [http://dx.doi.org/10.1142/S0219622020500285]

[11]   O.S. Albahri, J.R. Al-Obaidi, A.A. Zaidan, A.S. Albahri, B.B. Zaidan, M.M. Salih, A. Qays, K.A. Dawood, R.T. Mohammed, K.H. Abdulkareem, A.M. Aleesa, A.H. Alamoodi, M.A. Chyad, and C.Z. Zulkifli, "Helping doctors hasten COVID-19 treatment: Towards a rescue framework for the transfusion of best convalescent plasma to the most critical patients based on biological requirements via ml and novel MCDM methods", *Comput. Methods Programs Biomed.,* vol. 196, p. 105617, 2020.
       [http://dx.doi.org/10.1016/j.cmpb.2020.105617] [PMID: 32593060]

[12]   W.T. Li, J. Ma, N. Shende, G. Castaneda, J. Chakladar, J.C. Tsai, L. Apostol, C.O. Honda, J. Xu, L.M. Wong, T. Zhang, A. Lee, A. Gnanasekar, T.K. Honda, S.Z. Kuo, M.A. Yu, E.Y. Chang, M.R. Rajasekaran, and W.M. Ongkeko, "Using machine learning of clinical data to diagnose COVID-19: a systematic review and meta-analysis", *BMC Med. Inform. Decis. Mak.,* vol. 20, no. 1, p. 247, 2020.
       [http://dx.doi.org/10.1186/s12911-020-01266-z] [PMID: 32993652]

[13]   C.K. Monaghan, J.W. Larkin, S. Chaudhuri, H. Han, Y. Jiao, K.M. Bermudez, E.D. Weinhandl, I.A. Dahne-Steuber, K. Belmonte, L. Neri, P. Kotanko, J.P. Kooman, J.L. Hymes, R.J. Kossmann, L.A. Usvyat, and F.W. Maddux, "Machine Learning for Prediction of Patients on Hemodialysis with an Undetected SARS-CoV-2 Infection", *Kidney360,* vol. 2, no. 3, pp. 456-468, 2021.
       [http://dx.doi.org/10.34067/KID.0003802020] [PMID: 35369017]

[14]   X. Mei, "Artificial intelligence-enabled rapid diagnosis of COVID-19 patients", *medRxiv.* 2020.

[15]   L.P. Garcia, "Estimating underdiagnosis of COVID-19 with nowcasting and machine learning-experience from brazil", *medRxiv.* 2020.
       [http://dx.doi.org/10.1101/2020.07.01.20144402]

[16]   N-N. Sun, "A prediction model based on machine learning for diagnosing the early COVID-19 patients", *medRxiv.* 2020.
       [http://dx.doi.org/10.1101/2020.06.03.20120881]

[17]   M. Jamshidi, A. Lalbakhsh, J. Talla, Z. Peroutka, F. Hadjilooei, P. Lalbakhsh, M. Jamshidi, L.L. Spada, M. Mirmozafari, M. Dehghani, A. Sabet, S. Roshani, S. Roshani, N. Bayat-Makou, B. Mohamadzade, Z. Malek, A. Jamshidi, S. Kiani, H. Hashemi-Dezaki, and W. Mohyuddin, "Artificial intelligence and COVID-19: deep learning approaches for diagnosis and treatment", *IEEE Access,* vol. 8, pp. 109581-109595, 2020.
       [http://dx.doi.org/10.1109/ACCESS.2020.3001973] [PMID: 34192103]

[18]   S. Hassantabar, "CovidDeep: SARS-CoV-2/COVID-19 test based on wearable medical sensors and efficient neural networks", 2020.

[19]   M. Kukar, G. Gunčar, T. Vovko, S. Podnar, P. Černelč, M. Brvar, M. Zalaznik, M. Notar, S. Moškon, and M. Notar, "COVID-19 diagnosis by routine blood tests using machine learning", *Sci. Rep.,* vol. 11, no. 1, p. 10738, 2021.
       [http://dx.doi.org/10.1038/s41598-021-90265-9] [PMID: 34031483]

[20] F. Soares, "A novel specific artificial intelligence-based method to identify COVID-19 cases using simple blood exams", *medRxiv*. 2020.
[http://dx.doi.org/10.1101/2020.04.10.20061036]

[21] J.C. Gomes, "Optimizing the molecular diagnosis of COVID-19 by combining RT-PCR and a pseudo-convolutional machine learning approach to characterize virus DNA sequences", *bioRxiv*. 2020.
[http://dx.doi.org/10.1101/2020.06.02.129775]

[22] A. Imran, I. Posokhova, H.N. Qureshi, U. Masood, M.S. Riaz, K. Ali, C.N. John, M.D.I. Hussain, and M. Nabeel, "AI4COVID-19: AI enabled preliminary diagnosis for COVID-19 from cough samples via an app", *Informatics in Medicine Unlocked*, vol. 20, p. 100378, 2020.
[http://dx.doi.org/10.1016/j.imu.2020.100378] [PMID: 32839734]

[23] E. Fayyoumi, S. Idwan, and H. AboShindi, "Machine learning and statistical modelling for prediction of novel COVID-19 patients case study: jordan", *Int. J. Adv. Comput. Sci. Appl.*, vol. 11, no. 5, 2020.
[http://dx.doi.org/10.14569/IJACSA.2020.0110518]

[24] A.M.U.D. Khanday, S.T. Rabani, Q.R. Khan, N. Rouf, and M. Mohi Ud Din, "Machine learning based approaches for detecting COVID-19 using clinical text data", *International Journal of Information Technology*, vol. 12, no. 3, pp. 731-739, 2020.
[http://dx.doi.org/10.1007/s41870-020-00495-9] [PMID: 32838125]

[25] H. Al-Najjar, and N. Al-Rousan, "A classifier prediction model to predict the status of Coronavirus COVID-19 patients in South Korea", *Eur. Rev. Med. Pharmacol. Sci.*, vol. 24, no. 6, pp. 3400-3403, 2020.
[http://dx.doi.org/10.26355/eurrev_202003_20709] [PMID: 32271458]

[26] J. Sarkar, and P. Chakrabarti, "A Machine Learning Model Reveals Older Age and Delayed Hospitalization as Predictors of Mortality in Patients with COVID-19", *medRxiv*. 2020.
[http://dx.doi.org/10.1101/2020.03.25.20043331]

[27] L. Yan, H-T. Zhang, J. Goncalves, Y. Xiao, M. Wang, Y. Guo, C. Sun, X. Tang, L. Jing, M. Zhang, X. Huang, Y. Xiao, H. Cao, Y. Chen, T. Ren, F. Wang, Y. Xiao, S. Huang, X. Tan, N. Huang, B. Jiao, C. Cheng, Y. Zhang, A. Luo, L. Mombaerts, J. Jin, Z. Cao, S. Li, H. Xu, and Y. Yuan, "An interpretable mortality prediction model for COVID-19 patients", *Nat. Mach. Intell.*, vol. 2, no. 5, pp. 283-288, 2020.
[http://dx.doi.org/10.1038/s42256-020-0180-7]

[28] F.Y. Cheng, H. Joshi, P. Tandon, R. Freeman, D.L. Reich, M. Mazumdar, R. Kohli-Seth, M.A. Levin, P. Timsina, and A. Kia, "Using machine learning to predict icu transfer in hospitalized COVID-19 patients", *J. Clin. Med.*, vol. 9, no. 6, p. 1668, 2020.
[http://dx.doi.org/10.3390/jcm9061668] [PMID: 32492874]

[29] A.K. Das, S. Mishra, and S.S. Gopalan, "Predicting COVID-19 community mortality risk using machine learning and development of an online prognostic tool", *medRxiv*. 2020.
[http://dx.doi.org/10.1101/2020.04.27.20081794]

[30] Z. Yao, X. Zheng, Z. Zheng, K. Wu, and J. Zheng, "Construction and validation of a machine learning–based nomogram: A tool to predict the risk of getting severe coronavirus disease 2019 (COVID–19)", *Immun. Inflamm. Dis.*, vol. 9, no. 2, pp. 595-607, 2021.
[http://dx.doi.org/10.1002/iid3.421] [PMID: 33713584]

[31] A. Sehanobish, N.G. Ravindra, and D van Dijk, "Gaining Insight into SARS-CoV-2 Infection and COVID-19 severity using self-supervised edge features and graph neural networks", 2020.
[http://dx.doi.org/arXiv:2006.12971]

[32] X. Bai, "Predicting COVID-19 malignant progression with AI techniques", *medRxiv*. 2020.
[http://dx.doi.org/10.1101/2020.03.20.20037325]

[33] H. Yao, N. Zhang, R. Zhang, M. Duan, T. Xie, J. Pan, E. Peng, J. Huang, Y. Zhang, X. Xu, H. Xu, F. Zhou, and G. Wang, "Severity detection for the coronavirus disease 2019 (COVID-19) patients using a

machine learning model based on the blood and urine tests", *Front. Cell Dev. Biol.,* vol. 8, p. 683, 2020.
[http://dx.doi.org/10.3389/fcell.2020.00683] [PMID: 32850809]

[34]   J. Han, "An early study on intelligent analysis of speech under COVID-19: severity, sleep quality, fatigue, and anxiety", 2020.
[http://dx.doi.org/10.21437/Interspeech.2020-2223]

[35]   L. Yan, "Prediction of criticality in patients with severe COVID-19 infection using three clinical features: a machine learning-based prognostic model with clinical data in Wuhan", *medRxiv.* 2020.
[http://dx.doi.org/10.1101/2020.02.27.20028027]

[36]   F. Xu, X. Chen, X. Yin, Q. Qiu, J. Xiao, L. Qiao, M. He, L. Tang, X. Li, Q. Zhang, Y. Lv, S. Xiao, R. Zhao, Y. Guo, M. Chen, D. Chen, L. Wen, B. Wang, Y. Nian, and K. Liu, "Prediction of disease progression of COVID-19 based upon machine learning", *Int. J. Gen. Med.,* vol. 14, pp. 1589-1598, 2021.
[http://dx.doi.org/10.2147/IJGM.S294872] [PMID: 33953606]

[37]   H.S. Maghdid, K.Z. Ghafoor, A.S. Sadiq, K. Curran, D.B. Rawat, and Rabie, "A Novel AI-enabled Framework to Diagnose Coronavirus COVID 19 using Smartphone Embedded Sensors: Design Study", 2020.
[http://dx.doi.org/10.1109/IRI49571.2020.00033]

[38]   J.L. Izquierdo, J. Ancochea, and J.B. Soriano, "S. C.-19 R. Group, and others, "Clinical characteristics and prognostic factors for intensive care unit admission of patients With COVID-19: retrospective study using machine learning and natural language processing,", *J. Med. Internet Res.,* vol. 22, no. 10, p. e21801, 2020.
[http://dx.doi.org/10.2196/21801] [PMID: 33090964]

[39]   A. Onovo, "Using supervised machine learning and empirical bayesian kriging to reveal correlates and patterns of COVID-19 disease outbreak in sub-saharan africa: exploratory data analysis", *Soc. Sci. Res. Netw.,* 2020.
[http://dx.doi.org/10.2139/ssrn.3580721]

[40]   Z. Malki, E.S. Atlam, A.E. Hassanien, G. Dagnew, M.A. Elhosseini, and I. Gad, "Association between weather data and COVID-19 pandemic predicting mortality rate: Machine learning approaches", *Chaos Solitons Fractals,* vol. 138, p. 110137, 2020.
[http://dx.doi.org/10.1016/j.chaos.2020.110137] [PMID: 32834583]

[41]   A. Gupta, and A. Gharehgozli, "Developing a Machine Learning Framework to Determine the Spread of COVID-19", *Soc. Sci. Res. Netw.,* 2020.
[http://dx.doi.org/10.2139/ssrn.3635211]

[42]   M. Yadav, M. Perumal, and M. Srinivas, "Analysis on novel coronavirus (COVID-19) using machine learning methods", *Chaos Solitons Fractals,* vol. 139, p. 110050, 2020.
[http://dx.doi.org/10.1016/j.chaos.2020.110050] [PMID: 32834604]

[43]   D. Liu, "A machine learning methodology for real-time forecasting of the 2019-2020 COVID-19 outbreak using Internet searches, news alerts, and estimates from mechanistic models", 2020.
[http://dx.doi.org/arXiv:2004.04019v1]

[44]   F. Khmaissia, "An Unsupervised Machine Learning Approach to Assess the ZIP Code Level Impact of COVID-19 in NYC", 2020.
[http://dx.doi.org/arXiv:2006.08361v3]

[45]   I.G. Pereira, J.M. Guerin, A.G. Silva Júnior, G.S. Garcia, P. Piscitelli, A. Miani, C. Distante, and L.M.G. Gonçalves, "Forecasting COVID-19 Dynamics in Brazil: A Data Driven Approach", *Int. J. Environ. Res. Public Health,* vol. 17, no. 14, p. 5115, 2020.
[http://dx.doi.org/10.3390/ijerph17145115] [PMID: 32679861]

[46]   L.R. Kolozsvári, "Predicting the epidemic curve of the coronavirus (SARS-CoV-2) disease (COVID-

19) using artificial intelligence", *medRxiv.* 2020.
[http://dx.doi.org/10.1101/2020.04.17.20069666]

[47]   Z. Li, Y. Zheng, J. Xin, and G. Zhou, "A Recurrent Neural Network and Differential Equation Based Spatiotemporal Infectious Disease Model with Application to COVID-19", *medRxiv.* 2020.
[http://dx.doi.org/10.1101/2020.07.20.20158568]

[48]   A. Kapoor, "Examining COVID-19 Forecasting using Spatio-Temporal Graph Neural Networks", 2020.
[http://dx.doi.org/arXiv:2007.03113v1]

[49]   A. Chatterjee, M.W. Gerdes, and S.G. Martinez, "Statistical Explorations and Univariate Timeseries Analysis on COVID-19 Datasets to Understand the Trend of Disease Spreading and Death", *Sensors (Basel),* vol. 20, no. 11, p. 3089, 2020.
[http://dx.doi.org/10.3390/s20113089] [PMID: 32486055]

[50]   V.K.R. Chimmula, and L. Zhang, "Time series forecasting of COVID-19 transmission in Canada using LSTM networks", *Chaos Solitons Fractals,* vol. 135, p. 109864, 2020.
[http://dx.doi.org/10.1016/j.chaos.2020.109864] [PMID: 32390691]

[51]   C. Direkoglu, and M. Sah, "Worldwide and Regional Forecasting of Coronavirus (COVID-19) Spread using a Deep Learning Model", *medRxiv.* 2020.
[http://dx.doi.org/10.1101/2020.05.23.20111039]

[52]   F.M. Khan, and R. Gupta, "ARIMA and NAR based prediction model for time series analysis of COVID-19 cases in India", *Journal of Safety Science and Resilience,* vol. 1, no. 1, pp. 12-18, 2020.
[http://dx.doi.org/10.1016/j.jnlssr.2020.06.007]

[53]   L. Moftakhar, M. Seif, and M. S. Safe, "Exponentially Increasing Trend of Infected Patients with COVID-19 in Iran: A Comparison of Neural Network and ARIMA Forecasting Models", *Iran. J. Public Health,* vol. 49, no. no. Suppl 1, pp. 92-100, 2020.
[http://dx.doi.org/10.18502/ijph.v49iS1.3675]

[54]   T. Chakraborty, and I. Ghosh, "Real-time forecasts and risk assessment of novel coronavirus (COVID-19) cases: A data-driven analysis", *Chaos Solitons Fractals,* vol. 135, p. 109850, 2020.
[http://dx.doi.org/10.1016/j.chaos.2020.109850] [PMID: 32355424]

[55]   A.M. Javid, X. Liang, A. Venkitaraman, and Chatterjee, "Predictive Analysis of COVID-19 Time-series Data from Johns Hopkins University", 2020.
[http://dx.doi.org/10.48550/arXiv.2005.05060]

[56]   N. Poonia, and Azad, "Short-term forecasts of COVID-19 spread across Indian states until 1 May 2020", 2020.
[http://dx.doi.org/10.48550/arXiv.2004.13538]

[57]   V. Sangiorgio, and F. Parisi, "A multicriteria approach for risk assessment of COVID-19 in urban district lockdown", *Saf. Sci.,* vol. 130, p. 104862, 2020.
[http://dx.doi.org/10.1016/j.ssci.2020.104862] [PMID: 32536749]

[58]   Y. Ye, "α-Satellite: An AI-driven System and Benchmark Datasets for Hierarchical Community-level Risk Assessment to Help Combat COVID-19", 2020.
[http://dx.doi.org/10.48550/arXiv.2003.12232]

[59]   M.I. Uddin, S.A.A. Shah, and M.A. Al-Khasawneh, "A Novel Deep Convolutional Neural Network Model to Monitor People following Guidelines to Avoid COVID-19", *J. Sensors,* vol. 2020, pp. 1-15, 2020.
[http://dx.doi.org/10.1155/2020/8856801]

[60]   D. Yang, E. Yurtsever, V. Renganathan, K.A. Redmill, and Ü Özgüner, "A Vision-based Social Distancing and Critical Density Detection System for COVID-19", 2020.
[http://dx.doi.org/10.48550/arXiv.2007.03578]

[61]   N.S. Punn, S.K. Sonbhadra, S. Agarwal, and G Rai, "Monitoring COVID-19 social distancing with

person detection and tracking *via* fine-tuned YOLO v3 and Deepsort techniques", 2021.

[62]   N. Soures, "SIRNet: Understanding Social Distancing Measures with Hybrid Neural Network Model for COVID-19 Infectious Spread", 2020.
[http://dx.doi.org/10.48550/arXiv.2004.10376]

[63]   P. Khandelwal, A. Khandelwal, S. Agarwal, D. Thomas, N. Xavier, and Raghuraman, "Using Computer Vision to enhance Safety of Workforce in Manufacturing in a Post COVID World", 2020.
[http://dx.doi.org/10.48550/arXiv.2005.05287]

[64]   B. Qin, and D. Li, "Identifying Facemask-Wearing Condition Using Image Super-Resolution with Classification Network to Prevent COVID-19", *Sensors (Basel),* vol. 20, no. 18, p. 5236, 2020.
[http://dx.doi.org/10.3390/s20185236] [PMID: 32937867]

[65]   A.K.M.N. Islam, S. Laato, S. Talukder, and E. Sutinen, "Misinformation sharing and social media fatigue during COVID-19: An affordance and cognitive load perspective", *Technol. Forecast. Soc. Change,* vol. 159, p. 120201, 2020.
[http://dx.doi.org/10.1016/j.techfore.2020.120201] [PMID: 32834137]

[66]   R.F. Sear, N. Velasquez, R. Leahy, N.J. Restrepo, S.E. Oud, N. Gabriel, Y. Lupu, and N.F. Johnson, "Quantifying COVID-19 Content in the Online Health Opinion War Using Machine Learning", *IEEE Access,* vol. 8, pp. 91886-91893, 2020.
[http://dx.doi.org/10.1109/ACCESS.2020.2993967] [PMID: 34192099]

[67]   X. Song, J. Petrak, Y. Jiang, I. Singh, D. Maynard, and K. Bontcheva, "Classification aware neural topic model for COVID-19 disinformation categorisation", *PLoS One,* vol. 16, no. 2, p. e0247086, 2021.
[http://dx.doi.org/10.1371/journal.pone.0247086] [PMID: 33600477]

[68]   S. Shahsavari, P. Holur, T.R. Tangherlini, and V. Roychowdhury, "Conspiracy in the Time of Corona: Automatic detection of COVID-19 Conspiracy Theories in Social Media and the News", 2020.
[http://dx.doi.org/arXiv:2004.13783v1]

[69]   Y. Chen, W. Yang, and B Zhang, "Using Mobility for Electrical Load Forecasting During the COVID-19 Pandemic", 2020.
[http://dx.doi.org/10.48550/arXiv.2006.08826]

[70]   N. Norouzi, G. Zarazua de Rubens, S. Choupanpiesheh, and P. Enevoldsen, "When pandemics impact economies and climate change: Exploring the impacts of COVID-19 on oil and electricity demand in China", *Energy Res. Soc. Sci.,* vol. 68, p. 101654, 2020.
[http://dx.doi.org/10.1016/j.erss.2020.101654] [PMID: 32839693]

[71]   S Johnstone, "A Viral Warning for Change. COVID-19 Versus the Red Cross: Better Solutions Via Blockchain and Artificial Intelligence", *Soc. Sci. Res. Netw.,* 2020.
[http://dx.doi.org/10.2139/ssrn.3530756]

[72]   G. Chandra, R. Gupta, and N. Agarwal, "Role of Artificial Intelligence in Transforming the Justice Delivery System in COVID-19 Pandemic", *Int. J. Emerg. Technol.,* vol. 11, no. 3, pp. 344-350, 2020.

[73]   S. Bandyopadhyay, "Detection of Fraud Transactions Using Recurrent Neural Network during COVID-19", *Preprints.* 2020.
[http://dx.doi.org/10.20944/preprints202006.0368.v1]

[74]   T. Chen, L. Peng, X. Yin, J. Rong, J. Yang, and G. Cong, "Analysis of User Satisfaction with Online Education Platforms in China during the COVID-19 Pandemic", *Healthcare (Basel),* vol. 8, no. 3, p. 200, 2020.
[http://dx.doi.org/10.3390/healthcare8030200] [PMID: 32645911]

[75]   J. Ehrlich, and S. Ghimire, "COVID-19 countermeasures, Major League Baseball, and the home field advantage: Simulating the 2020 season using logistic regression and a neural network," *F1000Research*", 2020.
[http://dx.doi.org/10.12688/f1000research.23694.1]

[76]   A. Abdulla, B. Wang, F. Qian, T. Kee, A. Blasiak, Y.H. Ong, L. Hooi, F. Parekh, R. Soriano, G.G. Olinger, J. Keppo, C.L. Hardesty, E.K. Chow, D. Ho, and X. Ding, "Project identif.ai: harnessing artificial intelligence to rapidly optimize combination therapy development for infectious disease intervention", *Adv. Ther. (Weinh.),* vol. 3, no. 7, p. 2000034, 2020.
[http://dx.doi.org/10.1002/adtp.202000034] [PMID: 32838027]

[77]   S. Mohapatra, P. Nath, M. Chatterjee, N. Das, D. Kalita, P. Roy, and S. Satapathi, "Repurposing therapeutics for COVID-19: Rapid prediction of commercially available drugs through machine learning and docking", *PLoS One,* vol. 15, no. 11, p. e0241543, 2020.
[http://dx.doi.org/10.1371/journal.pone.0241543] [PMID: 33180803]

[78]   D. Morselli Gysi, Í. do Valle, M. Zitnik, A. Ameli, X. Gan, O. Varol, S.D. Ghiassian, J.J. Patten, R.A. Davey, J. Loscalzo, and A.L. Barabási, "Network medicine framework for identifying drug-repurposing opportunities for COVID-19", *Proc. Natl. Acad. Sci. USA,* vol. 118, no. 19, p. e2025581118, 2021.
[http://dx.doi.org/10.1073/pnas.2025581118] [PMID: 33906951]

[79]   X. Zeng, X. Song, T. Ma, X. Pan, Y. Zhou, Y. Hou, Z. Zhang, K. Li, G. Karypis, and F. Cheng, "Repurpose open data to discover therapeutics for COVID-19 using deep learning", *J. Proteome Res.,* vol. 19, no. 11, pp. 4624-4636, 2020.
[http://dx.doi.org/10.1021/acs.jproteome.0c00316] [PMID: 32654489]

[80]   A. López-Cortés, P. Guevara-Ramírez, N.C. Kyriakidis, C. Barba-Ostria, Á. León Cáceres, S. Guerrero, E. Ortiz-Prado, C.R. Munteanu, E. Tejera, D. Cevallos-Robalino, A.M. Gómez-Jaramillo, K. Simbaña-Rivera, A. Granizo-Martínez, G. Pérez-M, S. Moreno, J.M. García-Cárdenas, A.K. Zambrano, Y. Pérez-Castillo, A. Cabrera-Andrade, L. Puig San Andrés, C. Proaño-Castro, J. Bautista, A. Quevedo, N. Varela, L.A. Quiñones, and C. Paz-y-Miño, "In silico analyses of immune system protein interactome network, single-cell rna sequencing of human tissues, and artificial neural networks reveal potential therapeutic targets for drug repurposing against COVID-19", *Front. Pharmacol.,* vol. 12, p. 598925, 2021.
[http://dx.doi.org/10.3389/fphar.2021.598925] [PMID: 33716737]

[81]   R. Magar, P. Yadav, and A. Barati Farimani, "Potential neutralizing antibodies discovered for novel corona virus using machine learning", *Sci. Rep.,* vol. 11, no. 1, p. 5261, 2021.
[http://dx.doi.org/10.1038/s41598-021-84637-4] [PMID: 33664393]

[82]   "Sundar, Menaka, and Vinotha, "Artificial Intelligence Suggested Repositionable Therapeutics for Managing COVID-19: An Investigation with Machine Learning Algorithms and Molecular Structures," Res. Sq", 2020.
[http://dx.doi.org/10.21203/rs.3.rs-40988/v1]

[83]   M. Moskal, "Suggestions for second-pass anti-COVID-19 drugs based on the Artificial Intelligence measures of molecular similarity, shape and pharmacophore distribution", *ChemRxiv.* 2020.
[http://dx.doi.org/10.26434/chemrxiv.12084690.v2]

[84]   A. Zhavoronkov, "Potential Non-Covalent SARS-CoV-2 3C-like Protease Inhibitors Designed Using Generative Deep Learning Approaches and Reviewed by Human Medicinal Chemist in Virtual Reality", *ChemRxiv.* 2020.
[http://dx.doi.org/10.26434/chemrxiv.12301457.v1]

[85]   J. Stebbing, V. Krishnan, S. de Bono, G. Ottaviani, G. Casalini, P.J. Richardson, V. Monteil, V.M. Lauschke, A. Mirazimi, S. Youhanna, Y.J. Tan, F. Baldanti, A. Sarasini, J.A.R. Terres, B.J. Nickoloff, R.E. Higgs, G. Rocha, N.L. Byers, D.E. Schlichting, A. Nirula, A. Cardoso, and M. Corbellino, "Sacco baricitinib study groupmechanism of baricitinib supports artificial intelligence–predicted testing in covid–19 patients", *EMBO Mol. Med.,* vol. 12, no. 8, p. e12697, 2020.
[http://dx.doi.org/10.15252/emmm.202012697] [PMID: 32473600]

[86]   S. Ray, S. Lall, A. Mukhopadhyay, S. Bandyopadhyay, and A. Schönhuth, "Predicting potential drug targets and repurposable drugs for COVID-19 *via* a deep generative model for graphs", 2020.
[http://dx.doi.org/arXiv:2007.02338v1]

[87]   E. Ong, M.U. Wong, A. Huffman, and Y. He, "COVID-19 coronavirus vaccine design using reverse vaccinology and machine learning", *Front. Immunol.,* vol. 11, p. 1581, 2020.
[http://dx.doi.org/10.3389/fimmu.2020.01581] [PMID: 32719684]

[88]   G.K.M. Goh, A.K. Dunker, J.A. Foster, and V.N. Uversky, "A novel strategy for the development of vaccines for sars-cov-2 (COVID-19) and other viruses using ai and viral shell disorder", *J. Proteome Res.,* vol. 19, no. 11, pp. 4355-4363, 2020.
[http://dx.doi.org/10.1021/acs.jproteome.0c00672] [PMID: 33006287]

[89]   N.A. Brooks, A. Puri, S. Garg, S. Nag, J. Corbo, A.E. Turabi, N. Kaka, R.W. Zemmel, P.K. Hegarty, and A.M. Kamat, "The association of Coronavirus Disease-19 mortality and prior bacille Calmette-Guerin vaccination: a robust ecological analysis using unsupervised machine learning", *Sci. Rep.,* vol. 11, no. 1, p. 774, 2021.
[http://dx.doi.org/10.1038/s41598-020-80787-z] [PMID: 33436946]

[90]   H.M. Afify, and M.S. Zanaty, "Computational predictions for protein sequences of COVID-19 virus via machine learning algorithms", *Med. Biol. Eng. Comput.,* vol. 59, no. 9, pp. 1723-1734, 2021.
[http://dx.doi.org/10.1007/s11517-021-02412-z] [PMID: 34291385]

[91]   G.S. Randhawa, M.P.M. Soltysiak, H. El Roz, C.P.E. de Souza, K.A. Hill, and L. Kari, "Machine learning using intrinsic genomic signatures for rapid classification of novel pathogens: COVID-19 case study", *PLoS One,* vol. 15, no. 4, p. e0232391, 2020.
[http://dx.doi.org/10.1371/journal.pone.0232391] [PMID: 32330208]

[92]   R.K. Pathan, M. Biswas, and M.U. Khandaker, "Time series prediction of COVID-19 by mutation rate analysis using recurrent neural network-based LSTM model", *Chaos Solitons Fractals,* vol. 138, p. 110018, 2020.
[http://dx.doi.org/10.1016/j.chaos.2020.110018] [PMID: 32565626]

[93]   Savioli, "One-shot screening of potential peptide ligands on HR1 domain in COVID-19 glycosylated spike (S) protein with deep siamese network", 2020.

[94]   T.T. Nguyen, M. Abdelrazek, D.T. Nguyen, S. Aryal, D.T. Nguyen, and A. Khatami, "Origin of Novel Coronavirus (COVID-19): A Computational Biology Study using Artificial Intelligence", *bioRxiv.* 2020.
[http://dx.doi.org/10.1101/2020.05.12.091397]

CHAPTER 7

Case Study: Impact of Industry 4.0 and Its Impact on Fighting COVID–19

N. Hari Priya[1,*], **S. Rajeswari**[1] and **R. Gunavathi**[2]

[1] *Sree Saraswathi Thyagaraja College, Pollachi, Tamil Nadu, India*

[2] *Department of Data Science, CHRIST (Deemed to be University), Pune Lavasa Campus - The Hub of Analytics, Maharashtra 412112, India*

Abstract: The emerging development in industrial technology for automation and data sharing is known as Industry 4.0. It incorporates the Internet of Things, Cyber-physical systems, and Cloud computing, all of which contribute to the development of a "smart factory". Customers, distributors, vendors, and stakeholders in the supply chain would be capable of connecting and can exchange data easily through Industry 4.0. The COVID-19 pandemic is quickly spreading and posing a threat to people all over the world. Employment and activities in all markets have been disrupted, putting economies all over the world in serious jeopardy. To combat the pandemic, retailers will benefit from Industry 4.0 because it will help to mitigate the impact of identified risks. I4.0 executives were focused on gaining a competitive edge, rising efficiency, lowering prices, and, ensuring profitability as their primary aim was to enhance the productivity of business during the time before the COVID-19 crisis. Our Government has imposed new behavioral trends including social distancing, isolation and, lockdown. The Government needs additional financial resources to combat pandemics as a result of these actions, there has been a global economic slowdown. This chapter enlightens the significance and technologies of Industry 4.0, showing how those technologies and applications help in attaining a better society. It also explains how Industry 4.0 helps in accomplishing sustainable manufacturing and the management tactics it used to boost the company's efficiency, as well as the effects of COVID-19.

Keywords: Artificial Intelligence, Automation, Bigdata Analytics, COVID-19, Customer, Cloud Computing, Cybersecurity, Digital Manufacturing, Government, Global Economy, Industry4.0, Internet of Things, Manufacturers, Pandemic, Robots, Retailers, Supply Chain, Sustainable Manufacturing, Technologies, Virtualization.

---

[*] **Corresponding Author N. Hari Priya:** Sree Saraswathi Thyagaraja College, Pollachi, Tamil Nadu, India;
Tel: +91 94863 54525; E-mail: haripriyanarasimma@gmail.com

S. Vijayalakshmi, Naveen Chilamkurti, Savita, Rajesh Kumar Dhanaraj and Balamurugan Balusamy (Eds.)

INTRODUCTION

COVID-19 (coronavirus disease) pandemic has impacted nearly every country and had a substantial impact on healthcare facilities. The spread of COVID-19 wasc like wildfire posing a serious threat to 213 countries and territories all over the world [1]. This pandemic has disrupted employment and activities in all marketplaces, putting economies all over the world in significant peril [2]. The vision and implementation of a smart factory are made easier with Industry 4.0.

The German government first proclaimed Industry 4.0 as the start of the 4th industrial revolution during the Hannover Fair in 2011 [3]. The fourth industrial revolution is a novel degree of organization and control that encompasses the entire value chain of an item, from raw resources to production, distribution, assistance, and recycling. It is focused on the real-time intelligent management of all data available throughout the product and production system life cycle. The goal is to create a high level of product customization in a highly flexible mass-production environment. The basic idea of Industry 4.0 is to integrate machines, systems, and smart work pieces. Businesses create intelligent networks that can interact with each other independently along the whole value chain.

Industry 4.0's ultimate aim is to make manufacturing and allied industries more productive, quicker, and customer-centric, as well as to explore new business prospects and models beyond automation. Industry 4.0 promotes production efficiency by gathering information wisely, making sound judgments, and carrying them out without reluctance. Retailers will also benefit from Industry 4.0 to combat the pandemic because it will help to mitigate the impact of identified risks [4].

Industry 4.0 can transform the manufacturing industry to the next level. It also has the potential towards becoming a reality in which factory automation is widespread and factories are significantly more intelligent than it has been ever. Industry 4.0 aims to collect massive amounts of data from a variety of sources. The production planning tool is a crucial factor in translating acquired data into an actionable outcome that nourishes the networked supply chain inside the manufacturing environment.

The procedures for gathering and evaluating data will be made easier by utilizing the most current technologies. In Industry 4.0, the interoperability operational capability serves as a "connecting bridge" to ensure a stable manufacturing environment [5]. To deal with global difficulties and raise industrial levels, Industry 4.0 uses emerging technologies and the rapid progression of equipment and tools. By using technical expertise, production can run more quickly and smoothly with less downtime [6].

The drive to implement Industry 4.0 poses a wide range of technological obstacles, with significant implications across a wide variety of aspects of the manufacturing industry. As a result, developing a plan for all the actors of the complete value chain, as well as accomplishing an agreement on security issues and appropriate design before implementation begins, is critical.

COVID-19 and Technology

Various technologies have been employed to track the COVID-19 pandemic progression. All of these techniques and activities have been created in the hopes of slowing the spread of the disease. It has been used to keep an eye on public venues and patients, create new, effective vaccines, ensure the continuation of the education system and small and large businesses, and lessen the impact of quarantines on citizens, and relieve pressure on overburdened healthcare professionals [7].

The Enterprise Resource Planning (ERP) software is used at the corporate level. A business strategy, operations management, accounting, marketing and distribution, management of human resources, and other enterprise-wide marketing plans are all supported by ERP [8]. Artificial intelligence and drones have been performed to analyze public areas to determine whether or not social distancing was being reflected. Cloud-based platforms like Google Hangouts, Google Meet, and Zoom have now been deployed all around the world to make it simpler for employees to work and students to continue their education online. This chapter enlightens the significance and technologies of Industry 4.0, showing how those technologies and applications help in conquering a better society. It also explains how Industry 4.0 helps in accomplishing sustainable manufacturing and the management tactics it uses to boost the company's efficiency, as well as the COVID-19's effects.

CONCEPTUAL FRAMEWORK FOR INDUSTRY 4.0

Introduction

The use of emerging and rapidly evolving digital technology to tackle specific problems is referred to as digital transformation. It is rapidly becoming a top concern for enterprises around the world, and the planning phases have sped dramatically, particularly during the COVID-19 epidemic [9]. The core technology trends and design concepts have facilitated new production methods as a result of the digital transformation of manufacturing industries [10]. Manufacturing firms, service, and operational environments have been paying close attention to Industry 4.0. The focus is on manufacturing facilities, service integration systems, and supply chains that allow value-added networks to be deployed.

Industry 4.0 is a significant indication in the organization and control of the business supply chain that is used concurrently with the industrial revolution 4.0. Industry 4.0 is built on cyber-physical systems. They incorporate embedded systems, modern control systems, and an Internet address to connect and can be accessed through the use of the Internet of Things (IoT). After the commencement of rapid advances in the integration of production and digital technology, interlinked and smart products are being substantially reformed for value creation in industrial production and other sectors. To address the crucial interconnections between intelligent devices and smart processes, a conceptual framework is outlined in which the key components are explained.

It comes with several new features which have been uniquely distinguished among others and are listed here.

• More mechanisms in automation than during the third industrial revolution

• Cyber-physical systems that are empowered by IoT Technology are integrating the physical and digital worlds

• A transition from a centralized control system towards one in which smart products determine the production phases

• Control systems and data models will be in the closed-loop structure

According to [11], three characteristics should be considered for successful and efficient system adaption to Industry 4.0:

I. Horizontal Integration Through Value Chains

Horizontal integration refers to a company's expansion at the same stage of the supply chain, either within the same or a different industry. Internal expansion is one way for a firm to grow. This can happen when a retailer expands the number of products available in a given category. It is a competitive approach that can lead to cost savings, a competitive advantage, greater market share, and corporate growth. Strategic alliances aim for outcomes that increase resources, market share, expertise, and efficiency. The total benefit of horizontal integration is a rise in market dominance with only a minor cost of not being integrated.

II. Vertical Integration and Networked Production or Service Systems

Vertical integration entails the effective cross-linking and digitization of product lines at various organizational levels. As a result, vertical integration allows for a more flexible migration to a smart factory, allowing for the manufacturing of small batch sizes and tailored items while maintaining acceptable profit margins. Vertical integration includes purchasing and integrating in-house, a previously outsourced element of either the production or sales processes. The supply chain of a business usually starts with the acquisition of source (raw) materials from the supplier and terminates with the selling of the end product to customers.

III. End-to-End Value Chain Engineering

End-to-end engineering aids in product creation by digitally integrating supporting technologies considering customer needs, product design, service, and recycling. By eradicating the middleman, end-to-end processing can assist improve a company's efficiency and performance. End-to-end solutions are often more cost-effective in coping with complicated products or technologies.

Key Characteristics of an Industry 4.0 System

Interoperability: Sensors, machines, devices, and individuals can communicate with one another.

Information transparency: To examine the information, information systems generate a virtual replica of the actual environment using sensor data.

Decentralized decision-making: The competence of cyber-physical systems to make decisions and perform their roles as independently as possible.

Virtualization: The act of building a virtual instance instead of a physical version is referred to as virtualization. Virtualized machines are malware-resistant that are used to check for updates, perform software tests, and evaluate multiple configurations before delivering the final product.

Real-Time Response: Modern businesses have a new expectation and it is because technology has progressed to the point where sensors can feed data and algorithms in real-time. This significant data analysis yields instant results and allows for rapid solving of issues and maintenance planning.

The transition to Industry 4.0 is based on core technologies, such as Big data analytics, Artificial Intelligence, the Internet of Things, Cloud Computing, Cyber

Security, Autonomous Robots, Augmented Reality, Additive Manufacturing, Simulation, and Virtualization. Basic technologies including sensors, actuators, RFID *(Radio Frequency Identification)*, and RTLS *(Real-Time Locating Systems)* technologies, mobile applications and design concepts, should be used to facilitate the growth of these technologies [12].

Key Components

Big Data Analytics

Big data is an analytical approach that is well-suited for tracking and controlling the global spread of COVID 19. This system holds information on a large volume of virus-infected patients. This technique lays the foundation for more rapid and near-real-time analysis of decision-making. It facilitates the saving of lives and the rapid identification of effective medications [13]. Now there is a growth of a lot of data that can be collected and evaluated as systems have become more computerized and interconnected. The sheer volume of data is one of the difficulties, as it is tough to find the important facts and patterns that give rise to automated and efficient decisions when there's too much data. This is the point where the concept of Big data comes into the picture.

Big data analytics allows for the identification of a component's performance and operational constraints to prevent future challenges in productions and paves way for taking precautionary action. Analytics systems are advancing in line with the production industry as it moves toward Industry 4.0. To provide end-to-end (E2E) visibility, the Industry 4.0 supply chain employs advanced Big data analytics. Data is available in real-time to assist in quick decision-making and deliver insight into the whole production process, both within and beyond individual enterprises.

Artificial Intelligence

Recent innovations in Industrial AI have indicated the ability of digital technology to support manufacturers in overcoming the issues concerning the digital transition of Cyber systems *via* its data-driven forecasting and potential to aid decision-making in extremely complicated and multistage environments [14]. Business intelligence is strengthened by artificial intelligence, which is a crucial innovation for the world economy. For a smart factory with its Industry 4.0, artificial intelligence and its component machine learning are extremely necessary. Artificial intelligence has evolved in a swing in the way businesses operate, owing to a new type of human-machine interaction. It serves as a technique and methodology for developing products and solutions for applications based on industries, as well as a bridge between academic AI research and industry professionals [15].

Internet of Things (IoT)

The Internet of Things is a term used to describe computational technology incorporated in gadgets that could interact with devices and individuals over the world wide web. Through the networked world, Industry 4.0 has begun and it is used to describe a technological revolution that has been facilitated by the Internet of Things [16]. IoT is a critical feature of Industry 4.0 systems, it connects hardware components through a network to accumulate data for decision-making. IoT has great potential for obtaining real-time data, giving useful information, and low-cost predictive maintenance, also opening a new horizon of a data-driven method for adding value [17]. Embedded computers improve the quality and efficiency of the manufactured product. The use of networked devices and sensors across the supply chain is another facet of integration. The IoT is fully utilized in the Ir 4.0 production process for faster, flexible operations with significantly better accessibility and transparency.

Cloud Computing

Cloud Computing is the evolving technology that allows communication devices to transmit and store data and accomplish computations at third-party computing resources [18]. Performance benchmarking and Remote service are the applications areas in which the cloud is used and its significance in other industry sectors will grow exponentially. Cloud Computing stimulates a new trend of worldwide digital high-tech development in the Cyber-Physical System (CPS) of industry 4.0 by delivering computing resources such as centrally shared, flexible expansion. It helps to enlarge innovative business models and prospects for cloud services as well as cloud environment solutions including both Public and Private Cloud Infrastructure [19].

Cybersecurity

Cyber Security plays a crucial role in preventing businesses from losing their competitive edge in the era of Industry 4.0 [20]. Information security becomes crucially influential as we move from closed systems as a result of increased integration from the Cloud and Internet of Things. The effective implementation of a completely modern and computerized production workflow, utilizing all of the beneficial effects of a connected environment, is made possible by accuracy and protection. The supply chain has become extremely fragile as a result of the rising dependency on interlinked gadgets and data. The first stage for distribution network executives is to set up reliable collaboration and communication standards which could be accomplished throughout the organization. The protocols used need to be supplemented and backed by strict identity network access to secure all production processes and significant manufacturing systems. As a result, cybersecurity must always be a top priority for the enterprise.

Autonomous Robots

Autonomous robots are still in their development stage. This is largely due to the high cost of the technology and the limited abilities of autonomous robots. However, as the abilities and the costs of robots are getting increased, this technological innovation will become extremely important in the smart manufacturing production process. It has been predicted by experts that autonomous robots would communicate directly with one another and also with people shortly. When combined with machine learning algorithms, these robots will transform the supply chain, making it more responsive, interconnected, and reactive.

Augmented Reality

Manufacturers can increase efficiency, quality, and security by using real-time data given by augmented reality systems. AR incorporates all of the advantages of automated evaluation, improved accuracy, and non-destructive fault analysis also incorporating human skill and judgment at every step. The competence of industrial robotic systems is expanding rapidly, and an increased collaborative interaction is expected. Operators must operate in a secure atmosphere that allows them to have a belief in robots. The integration of AR into the industrial arena is pertinent because it enhances interaction in the design and development of a product. It aids in the earlier detection and avoidance of design faults and it decreases the number of prototypes to be built and saves time and money for firms [21].

BENEFITS OF ADOPTING INDUSTRY 4.0

Industry 4.0 entails the amalgamation of manufacturing facilities, supply chains, and service operations to create value-added networks [22]. Industry 4.0 offers traditional manufacturing firms a new business model and even a potential concept for value creation [23]. It includes all of the additional automation and digitalization that businesses are now doing to optimize their cycle time and "link" all of the many job parts into a cohesive digital ecosystem. Without sacrificing quality, cost, or speed, Industry 4.0 will provide far higher flexibility and mobility in manufacturing. As a result, the company will be able to innovate more quickly and generate more income.

The following are some of the fundamental benefits of incorporating Industry 4.0 in the manufacturing sector:

1. The Internet of Things (IoT) is being used in manufacturing

2. Advanced maintenance and monitoring capabilities ensure greater business continuity

3. Improvement in agility

4. The creation of new economic models and innovative capabilities

5. Real-time tracking, IoT-enabled performance improvement, and Cobots all contribute to higher-quality products

6. As a result of automation and optimization, productivity has been amplified

Due to the extreme benefits that Industry 4.0 technologies provide; the ROI prospects are considerable. This comprises automation, production oversight, machine-to-machine communication, and decision-making systems. The benefits of Industry 4.0, which incorporate improved production and efficiency, enhanced flexibility and agility, and enhanced profitability are given below.

Increase Efficiency

Firms can make faster judgments and maintain high efficiency with fewer people and greater automation. Automation also helps to maintain a high level of quality, which helps to increase efficiency. The most significant advantage of Industrial IoT is that it allows firms to automate and thereby improve their operational efficiency. Robotics, automated and computerized technology can increase production and assist firms to streamline their processes by working more effectively. Physical machinery has been linked to software through sensors that will periodically check performance. As a result, manufacturers can gain a deeper insight into the working performance of specific pieces of equipment.

Collaborative Work and Enhanced Knowledge Sharing

Manufacturing processes, business systems, and departments can communicate with Industry 4.0 technologies regardless of geographic location, platform, time zone, or any other circumstance. This allows knowledge gained by a sensor in one factory, to be shared throughout the firm. Without any human intervention, this can be done automatically either through machine-to-machine or system-t--system. Data from a single sensor can immediately improve many production lines situated anywhere on the globe.

Better Customer Experience

Industry 4.0 provides chances to improve customer service and improve the consumer experience. Problems are rapidly fixed with the automated tracking and tracing functionality. Furthermore, challenges with product availability will be resolved, the quality of the product will get increased, and the buyers will have more options.

Reduces Costs

Although Industry 4.0 will demand initial expenditures, costs will be reduced once intelligence is incorporated into processes and products. Costs will be reduced as a result of the speed and capacity to handle a large mix smoothly. Industry 4.0 technology, such as automation, data management, and systems integration will substantially reduce production costs. The following are the primary factors that have resulted in lower costs:

- More efficient use of resources

- Machine and production line downtime is reduced.

- Manufacturing is much more efficient.

- Overall operational costs are lower.

- Waste of resources and products is minimized.

- Products have fewer quality difficulties.

DESIGN PRINCIPLES

Industry 4.0 is a paradigm that is transforming the way people live and work. Artificial intelligence and smart devices have advanced technologies that are part of daily life for both consumers and enterprises. Manufacturers can build smarter factories using Industry 4.0, allowing them to customize products more readily to different customers. Each of the design principles outlined contains the premise of offering a sustainable solution to any enterprise experiencing I4.0 transformation.

Interoperability

The potential for systems to function together by readily accessing as well as utilizing each other's features is referred to as interoperability [24]. Organizational, technological, application and semantic integration are the four generic levels of integration in interoperability frameworks [25]. The capability of machines, sensors, gadgets, and individuals to build relationships with one another through the use of the Internet of Things is explored in this fundamental principle (IoT). It establishes a link between data-generating nodes that can be accessed and controlled at any time and from any location. The ability of technology to deliver enhanced information for decision-making is the focus of this idea. It ensures that the numerous innovations, parts, and agents in Industry 4.0 are seamlessly integrated across business ecosystems [26].

Virtualisation

Virtualization permits a "digital shadow" of the warehouse to be generated electronically by integrating sensor data obtained from observing physical tools and materials with virtual simulation models. It is used to minimize the cost of hardware and the number of physical resources necessary in industries that do not rely on massive equipment and machines. Virtual data can enhance the view of decision-makers by allowing them to monitor equipment conditions in real-time and detect limitations in the system [27].

Decentralisation

Decentralization refers to a cyber-physical system's (CPS) ability to commit activities and make decisions on its own. It is supported by technologies including smart actuators, IoT, sensors, CPS, artificial intelligence, and additional technologies that can interact, exchange information, and control all production processes. Hence systems would be sensitive to small changes, making the process of reconsidering easier, more adaptable, and even presenting alternative solutions [28].

Real-Time Capability

A capability that can gather, transmit, examine, monitor, and exchange data in real-time is referred to as real-time capability [31]. Real-time processing and analysis of data can assist in enhancing decision-making, tracking manufacturing processes, detecting anomalies, recognizing optimization possibilities, and even identifying micro trends. Big data analytics and cloud computing could be an incredible platform for real-time data processing and analysis, as well as for integrating analytics into the system and thereby identifying obstacles in the supply chain [29]. Imaging systems like scanners, bots, Radio Frequency Identification (RFID), and other interconnected IoT devices are emerging technologies that could acquire real-time data.

Service Orientation

Customer-centric production is required as people and intelligent devices have to be able to interact effectively *via* the services provided by the internet to produce products that satisfy customers' needs. Nowadays, instead of merely delivering products, the new company strategy requires the production of new holistic solutions for customers. As a result, firms must concentrate not just on product development but also on customer service which can be accomplished through the incorporation of people with smart tools using the Internet of Service (IoS). IoS platform integrates services provided by individuals and smart systems both in and out of the firm. It adds value by allowing companies to stay up to date and establish new revenue streams through the proficient integration of all stakeholders [30].

Modularity

The potential of smart factories to adapt themselves to the new market trend is crucial in a dynamic market. An average firm would certainly take a week to research the market and adjust its output accordingly in a typical instance. Individual modules of modular systems can be replaced or expanded to meet the changing requirements. As a result, in the occurrence of seasonal variations or changes in product qualities, modular systems could be quickly altered [31].

ROLE OF INDUSTRY 4.0 IN FACILITATING THE PROMOTION OF SUSTAINABLE MANUFACTURING

Sustainable Manufacturing

Sustainable manufacturing is defined as the combination of systems and processes that can generate high-quality services and products with more sustainable resources while also being safer for customers and employees in which they operate, and mitigating social and environmental impacts across the whole of their entire life cycle [32].

Technologies of I4.0 are projected to play an important role in industrial manufacturing sustainability. The major goal of sustainability is to build and produce manufacturing methods and products that have no negative environmental impact and can attain 100% flawless product recyclability. While technical developments enable product and process development, digital technologies must be fused with sustainability to achieve sustainable development. As a result, manufacturers are concentrating their efforts upon these convergences to reap the full benefits of Industry 4.0, which would be sustainable production. In terms of the social aspect of sustainable manufacturing, I4.0 aids in the development of quality services and better products, which benefits society as a whole.

The creativity and novelty of technological growth contribute to a better global environment by generating a green, resource-secure, and progressive economy. In addition, technologies like machine learning, artificial intelligence, data analytics, IoT, and others can be utilized to construct, extend, and analyze the efficacy of sustainable development [33].

The significance of Industry 4.0 technologies and their Benefits in Promoting the Sustainable Manufacturing

I. IoT and IIoT

The Internet of Things (IoT) and the Industrial Internet of Things (IIoT) are the most important digital transformation technologies. It links manufacturing areas with sensors and gadgets that communicate with one another. The Internet of Things (IoT) covers a broad range of enterprises and users. IoT technology can be used by consumers as well as experts in fields such as healthcare, business, and government. IIoT technology is only employed by professionals in the industrial area in industrial settings. Consumers of IIoT and IoT technologies seem to have slightly distinct objectives in mind. The goal of IoT implementation is usually to boost efficiency, improve health & wellbeing, and improve user experiences. The first two aims are usually the focus of IIoT, which is less user-centric.

Benefits

• Unwanted production stages are avoided

• Management of waste and inventory

• Energy consumption is monitored and managed

• By delivering real-time alerts, it increases the safety of both the device and the operator

II. *Autonomous Robots and Cobots*

Mechanical equipment that works alongside humans with a high level of autonomy. When robotics is used correctly, it results in an evident increase in a company's activities. It has a good impact on everyday operations, simplifies the entire assembly workflow process, and even aids in the production of food. Many professions are hazardous or contain large amounts of content that can harm people. Due to their dexterity and strong machine learning capabilities, robots, on the other hand, are avoiding making those flaws [34].

Benefits

• Reduction in the workload of employees

• Creating smart workshops close to the client's site

III. *Virtualization*

Combining digital and real-world industrial content to create mixed reality is known as virtualization. Virtualization can be applied to a network, a server, or a single platform. It lets to split a single desktop into two virtual machines or operate numerous sessions for multiple persons or tasks on the same server at the same time as like done by cloud computing applications. A virtualized cloud environment will do tasks that are radically different from those performed by a virtualized corporate system, and it will perform tasks that are even more distant from those performed by a virtualized embedded system.

Benefits

• Maintenance and training can both be done remotely

• Maintenance activities can be managed remotely to save cost

IV. Additive Manufacturing

Additive manufacturing allows for the creation of customized items with cheaper capital costs, reduced turnaround time, less energy consumption during manufacturing, and less wastage of materials. It may be used to construct complicated parts and allows businesses to lower inventory, develop on-demand products, create reduced specialized production settings, and even shorten supply chains. To create a prototype, sequential depositions of different materials are used.

Benefits

• A decline in waste production

• Enhanced product customization

• The development time of the product will be reduced drastically

V. System Integration

In system integration, by integrating the value chain, a larger value network is created. System integration enhances the utility of a network by combining components and software applications to provide additional features. Industry 4.0, the fourth iteration of Industrialization that combines computers and robotics technology to optimize production efficiency, is now underway around the world.

Benefits

• Improved transparency and waste reduction

• There is no interruption in communication with the stakeholders

INDUSTRY 4.0 AND COVID–19

Social distancing has been recognized as the best feasible defensive technique against the COVID-19 outbreak due to the deficiency of any specific treatment protocol. Governments all over the world have enforced lockdowns due to the necessity for social distance. The rapid spread of COVID-19 has led countries to prohibit the movement of a large number of commodities across national borders, putting global trade flow in jeopardy [35].

COVID-19 is hastening the adoption of technologies of Industry 4.0 such as IoT and edge computing. Industry 4.0 technologies were already having a significant impact on the transition of manufacturers in the world before COVID-19. COVID-19 hasn't put us all on a new path, instead, it has sped up the progress. A few years ago, merely 20.7% of manufacturing businesses when interviewed classified them as 'highly prepared' to face the developing business strategies of Industry 4.0 [36].

Geolocation is yet another Ir 4.0 technology that is contributing to this pandemic-driven shift. Sensor data can assist businesses in determining the location of specific assets at any given time. They can change or adapt their business procedures based on this information. Industry 4.0 features modern manufacturing and informational technology to meet the personalized needs of various humans in several regions in a shorter time. In the services and manufacturing sectors, these technologies enable wireless communication to improve automation [13].

Machines in Industry 4.0 enterprises are assisted by wireless technology and sensors. These sensors are integrated into a system that can observe and monitor the entire manufacturing process as well as make choices on its own. To address the COVID-19 pandemic crisis, Industry 4.0 employs smart manufacturing techniques to produce necessary disposable products.

Industry 4.0 is based on the conception or formation of workplaces, smart services, and products interconnected through the Internet-of-Things (IoT) and Cyber-Physical Systems, which are having a significant impact on manufacturing [37]. The possibilities could lead to the value chains and their associated regions' long-term sustainability. By replacing the human workforce with robots, Industry 4.0 might potentially create issues such as societal disparities pertaining to the status of the individual in the labor force.

The popularity of distance learning has increased in recent years. This teaching approach and knowledge transfer save money and improve students' transportation dynamics, but it is related to social distance as well as the consumption of computational resources. As IR 4.0 transforms every enterprise into a tech corporation, privacy problems are a rising issue, as food, commercial, and financial businesses are going digital and accumulating a huge volume of personal information of their consumers [38].

What Effect did COVID-19 have on the Global Economy in 2020?

Manufacturing pertains to the GDP of nations and plays a significant part in their development as manufacturing industries are a significant contributing factor to the world economy [39]. The economic lockdown imposed to limit the spread of the virus has caused a significant slowdown in growth in economies all across the world. As a consequence, there has been a supply shock, which has led to a decline in output, labor, and demand. With the more serious threat of the pandemic, the Indian economy had been experiencing severe structural challenges and a slowdown, which have likely faded into the backdrop.

COVID-19 is causing unprecedented and rising human expenditures around the world for protecting people's lives and allowing medical systems to manage essential quarantine and large-scale closures to stop the disease from spreading. As a result, the financial operations are being impacted by the health crisis. The worldwide economy is expected to fall to 3% in the year 2020 as a result of the COVID-19 pandemic, which is even worse than the global catastrophe in the year 2008–2009. The effect on India's actual and speculative economic sectors is far worse than it was during the 2008 financial crisis. The nation is now facing plenty of issues, mainly economic and medical crises and commodities price collapses [40].

The greatest effect is anticipated to be on domestic consumption, as people avoid outdoor places by preference, but also due to government-imposed limitations on mobility and transportation to prevent disease transmission. Most production facilities have shut down as a result of the propagation of COVID-19 and most countries are experiencing labor shortages as a result of the virus proliferation.

The outbreak has claimed many lives around the world, and it poses an unanticipated threat to food supply, public health and, the workplace. Furthermore, social isolation, contradictory communications from officials, and a continual state of ambiguity have all been identified as major contributors to emotional discomfort and negatively impacting mental health and social well-being.

The Impact of the COVID-19 epidemic in Daily Life

The COVID-19 disaster has drastically altered people's lives and careers. COVID-19 had a rapid impact on our daily lives, enterprises, and global access to markets. Because the virus spreads aggressively from person to person, early detection of the illness is critical for controlling its spread. The majority of countries have reduced their product manufacturing. Businesses of millions of people are at risk of going out of business. Probably half of the world's largest 3.3 billion workers are in danger of losing their careers. The cause of this ailment has an impact on a variety of sectors and industries. COVID-19 has a wide range of effects in everyday life and has far-reaching implications. These could be classified into several categories:

A). Healthcare

• Diagnosing the disease, isolation, and treating suspicious or confirmed cases pose challenges.

• The present health care system is under a lot of strain.

• Patients suffering from different diseases and health issues are widely ignored.

• Health professionals and other healthcare providers are overburdened, putting them at risk.

• Medical stores are heavily burdened and there exists a breakdown in the pharmaceutical supply chain.

• High-level protection is required.

B). Economic

• Manufacturing of essential products and goods have been decreased

• Losses in business on a national and global scale.

• In the market, there is a lack of cash flow and the revenue growth rates have declined significantly.

C). Social

• The service industry is unable to deliver adequate service.

• Large-scale sporting events and championship contests had been cancelled or postponed.

• Eliminating regional and global travel as well as service cancellations.

• Cultural, spiritual, and social occasions are disrupted, causing immense anxiety in the community.

• Distancing ourselves from our friends and family members.

• Closure of entertainment venues such as shopping malls, sports clubs, gyms, theatres, and pools.

• Exams are being postponed and cancelled.

IMPACTS OF INDUSTRY 4.0 IN FIGHTING AGAINST THE COVID-19

The COVID-19 outbreak spread over the Western world in March 2020. Many nations lowered their economy and imposed strict limitations to prevent the progression of the disease. The world's second-largest nation with a population of about 1.34 billion, surviving in India is facing challenges in preventing the spread of severe respiratory disorder among its citizens. To deal with the current outbreak, a variety of strategies, including statistical techniques, computational modeling, and quantitative assessments, as well as the invention of a novel treatment, would be essential.

The Government of India took essential and stringent measures to combat the deadly virus, including deploying health checkpoints across country borders to determine whether persons arriving into the nation are infected with the virus. Many countries have implemented rescue missions and surveillance measures for citizens seeking to leave China.

India trades with its neighboring countries, including Nepal, Bangladesh, Myanmar, Bhutan, China, and Pakistan. Indian regional trade totalled over $12 billion in the financial year 2017–18, accounting for about 1.56% of the country's total worldwide trade of $769 billion. The spread of such infections will have a substantial negative impact on the Indian economy [41]. Instability in health service delivery and periodic vaccinations, few people seeking medical care, and budget constraints for non-COVID-19 treatments, deaths from several other causes are believed to have increased as a result of the pandemic. In March 2021, the second "pulse survey" by WHO with 135 countries revealed widespread disruptions over a complete year into the epidemic, with nearly 90% of nations indicating more interruptions to key health services.

COVID-19's Effects on Mental Health

The COVID-19 outbreak and the consequent economic downturn have created a negative impact on the mental health of people and created new difficulties for those who already suffer from depression [42]. These acute Covid pandemics are widely established to pose harm to mental health. Similarly, two recent studies indicated that COVID-19 has a consistently negative influence on mental health, with 16–18% of individuals exhibiting a symptom of depression [43]. It focuses on groups that were more vulnerable to poor mental health or substance misuse effects during the epidemic, such as young individuals, those who had lost their jobs, families, racial minorities, and key employees.

Mass unemployment is linked to greater depression, stress, discomfort, and lack of self-esteem, as well as increased rates of substance use sickness and suicide, as shown by former research on economic downturns. Adults in families with the loss of employment or lower salaries reported significantly higher levels of mental disorder symptoms than those in households without a job or with financial losses during the pandemic.

A STUDY ON THE MANUFACTURING INDUSTRIES

COVID-19's outburst is the most significant event that has occurred in 2020 as of now. It has already affected 12.5 million people around the world and is still increasing steadily, despite the nation's attempt to develop a vaccine. COVID-19 spread quickly as a pandemic, affecting millions of people as well as global commercial processes. Owing to the COVID-19's additive effect, the vast majority of manufacturers consider Industry 4.0 to be a critical component of their strategy for adapting to the change as well as for serving their communities in a better way.

Many organizations used Industry 4.0 technologies to respond to the epidemic, but perhaps the crisis is placing the future and sustainability of digital operations under additional strain. Enterprises across industries, particularly the manufacturing sector are facing uncertainty and interruptions as a result of the global pandemic. Some manufacturers have witnessed a decrease in demand, while others have seen an increase in demand, transferring or relocating operations to fulfill demand or create new products. Manufacturers should encourage growth by employing the most skilled and talented professionals inflexible in line with emerging, while reducing downtime, limiting risk, and safeguarding intellectual property, to be competitive in today's overall global marketplaces.

The widespread COVID-19 outbreak has pushed our world into disrupting cultural, societal, and business conventions. It demonstrated the significance of contingency planning in the supply chain breakdown. It also emphasized that the pace of the 4th industrial revolution is more crucial than it has ever been, as the industry prepares for another transformation into what could propel the next era of manufacturing ahead.

Over the last year, businesses around various countries have faced several most challenging issues in the supply chain, ranging from trade conflicts to natural calamities, and currently facing a worldwide crisis. Companies have never faced complexity as they do now as a result of macro conditions. The problems have revealed a key aspect of today's supply chain which is "they can't thrive without flexibility". Industry 4.0 is required to transform manufacturing due to the increased impact of macroeconomic indicators on production and supply chains, as well as the capacity to onshore manufacturing while preserving total cost and excellence also by enhancing reliability. Industry 4.0 will aid in the development of a sustainable and innovative business strategy.

Challenges Confronted by Manufacturing Industries in the Year 2020

1. Global competitive pressures: To assist in managing the risk in production processes amidst disruptive also during difficult times, manufacturers must focus on providing a prominent level of digital customer experience and enhance their efforts towards strategic initiatives that build scalability and agility. The high demand here is to offer items more quickly and for less money while retaining quality.

2. Increasing product and supply chain complexity: Organizations require information systems to assist them in navigating this complexity across the product lifecycle, from design to supply chain and production operations. It leads to the development of sophisticated products with complex manufacturing procedures.

3. Change: Supply chain risks are foreseeable in a dynamic international market. The manufacturing business is continually changing in terms of procurement and freight logistics, particularly as an effect of the COVID-19 outbreak. Industrial supply chains will have to become more tolerant of future catastrophes.

4. Technology innovation evolves at an incredible speed: Most manufacturing businesses are striving to keep up with the increasing advancement of technological innovation, which includes everything from sensing devices to automated robotics, artificial intelligence, cloud computing, and IoT.

To overcome all these challenges, manufacturers need to take five essential and foundational steps to leverage the benefits of Industry 4.0 technologies. By following all of these measures, an organization can overcome the aforementioned issues by reducing downtime and increasing the production of the business.

• Selecting the appropriate infrastructure

• Maintaining a strong business continuity plan

• Establishing a secure connection

• Consider hiring expert assistance like outsourcing

• Always keeping everything safe.

ROLE OF DIGITAL MANUFACTURING IN THE COVID-19 ERA

The COVID-19 epidemic has hastened the digital manufacturing process. Companies that formerly considered this as an alternative, now see it as an immediate requirement for sustaining their business in the current scenario. This is especially suitable for older establishments that have been undergoing renovations for several years. Due to the extremely lingering COVID-19 conflict, the industry appears to have expedited its transition to Industry 4.0 which states the quick pace of digitization in the manufacturing industry.

Technology has altered the way how businesses were carried out over the last several decades, but the industrial sector has been extremely slow to close the gap. Manufacturers are continuously using technologies like predictive analytics, IoT and, artificial intelligence to achieve success in their supply chain operations in recent times.

Industries would employ connectivity, automation, sophisticated analytics, and advanced engineering as part of the fourth industrial revolution. Based on the surveys and assessments, these improvements are assisting businesses in improving efficiency, optimizing speed to market, developing innovative business models, and enabling high degrees of product customization. Manufacturers have been able to install robots alongside humans on production floors especially with the emergence of 'Cobots.'

COVID-19 has driven our country's manufacturers to expedite the implementation of digital manufacturing technologies. According to the report of KPMG, companies in India have surpassed their worldwide counterparts on a wide range of issues, incorporating new business development and workforce paradigms. This tendency will be accelerated by an influx of foreign investment into India's digital sector.

OBJECTIVE OF THE STUDY

Industry 4.0 seems to be the most notable chapter of the Industrial Revolution, focusing primarily on industrial automation, real-time data collection, intelligent systems, and network connectivity, with the major purposes of increasing productivity, enhancing readily accessible work schedules, and rising the organizational ability to compete. Through its basic features of digitization, connectivity, paperless work, and optimal web access. The utilization of Industry 4.0 to enhance manufacturing and productivity improvement, as well as to handle supply chain difficulties, is an emerging topic of study. The rate of acceptance, however, varies for every company. The major bottlenecks to Industry 4.0 implementation are a lack of a defined vision, plan, strategy, and a structured road map.

Companies were hit three times by a global health epidemic, an economic catastrophe, and racial conflict during COVID-19. People and product supply chains are disrupted and organizations are now taking a hard look at their supply chain operations in the hopes of avoiding more interruptions that could lead to the failure of certain businesses. Many businesses have accelerated their migration to Industry 4.0 which is the continuing automation of conventional manufacturing and production activities utilizing modern and smart technologies thereby incorporating digital manufacturing techniques. Industry 4.0 is indeed a great asset in today's modern shifting work culture following the CORONA epidemic. It also advises on the use of industrial automation machines that communicate with customers in real-time.

Digital manufacturing aims to utilize technology to reduce the impact of factors both internally and externally while building a production process that aids in achieving profitability. Digital manufacturing would continue its speed of progress as long as the technology evolves. The current worldwide pandemic shows flaws in the global supply chain that can be eliminated with digital manufacturing which can respond immediately thereby ensuring performance and consistency.

This chapter deals with the case study on the impact of Industry 4.0 in fighting against COVID-19. The main objective of this case study is to identify the role of digital manufacturing during this pandemic and how it aids in product development and disruptions occurring in supply chain management. For the case study, a manufacturing industry known as "PROTO LABS" is chosen and for the development of a quick prototype and on-demand production, Protolabs serves as the fastest digital manufacturing platform. With automated and computerized 3D printing, fabrication of sheet metal, CNC machining, and injection molding capabilities, the technology-enabled enterprise could create innovative components and assemblies possibly in a short period. Their digital manufacturing method allows for quicker swiftness to market, lowers the cost for development and production, and lowers the risk throughout the entire life cycle of the product. The firm surveyed to learn further about their customers' experiences and perspectives in the event of the crisis and the survey was sent to nearly 105 customers among 12 industries by last year during June and July. Insights obtained from engineers, supply chain managers, and designers could be able to analyze how customers use digital manufacturing not only to survive during this crisis but also how they use it to prosper in the future.

ANALYSIS AND FINDINGS

Based on the survey conducted by Protolabs [44], COVID-19 emphasized the necessity of manufacturing to strengthen the resources. However, the organizations that gain the competitive advantage will use the knowledge gained from the crisis to create flexible, robust, and modernized supply chains that drive innovation as the speed and flexibility are provided by digital manufacturing. The most essential benefits that a company could get from its supplier are quality, speed, and reliability. If these supplier characteristics were never more crucial so it is the point where digital manufacturing comes into play.

As per the report, COVID-19 has exposed flaws in the supply chain. To reduce costs, the traditional supply chain which is oriented on negotiation, pricing, and globalization relies on procuring stock levels and suppliers from all around the world. This strategy holds up cash flow and flopped for many firms during COVID-19. The Protolabs survey predicted that nearly two-thirds of enterprises have been harmed by supplier delays, while more than 50% have been impacted by demand shifts which are shown in Fig. (**1**).

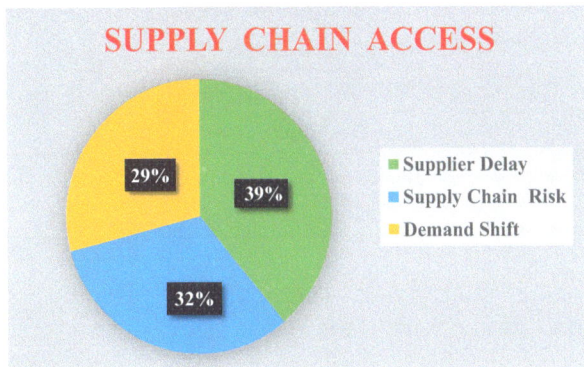

SUPPLY CHAIN ACCESS

29%　39%　32%

- Supplier Delay
- Supply Chain Risk
- Demand Shift

Fig. (1). Supply chain and access disruption (Source [44]).

Hindrances Faced Due to Work from Home Mode in Terms of Productivity

• In the initial days of the epidemic, widespread work-from-home orders worsened the dual effect on market forces.

• During June, a large proportion of those surveyed reported that approximately half of their employees still were working remotely

• Inaccessibility in getting the appropriate tools to carry out the process to be fully productive.

• Employees were also blocked off from people, making it difficult for them to collaborate with their co-workers.

Impacts Faced During COVID-19

A supplier is an individual or organization that sells a product or provides a service to another enterprise. A supplier's job in a firm is to offer high-quality products and services from a manufacturer to a retailer or distributor for resale at a reasonable price. In the pandemic, situation customers faced a lot of issues and their impacts are tabulated in Table **1**.

Table 1. Impacts faced by customers during COVID-19. (Source [44]).

Impacts Faced During COVID-19	Results
Supplier delays	74%
Using new manufacturing suppliers	19%
Delay in product launches	47%
A downturn in the new product development timeline	38%
Overall product funding reductions	38%
A decline in product innovation	38%
Working on COVID-19 specific products	29%
Uplifted manufacturing costs	12%
Working with different customers	9%
Others	8%

Certain factors are considered important in a supplier by a customer and the factors are presented along with their percentage score in Fig. (**2**).

PROMINENT FACTORS

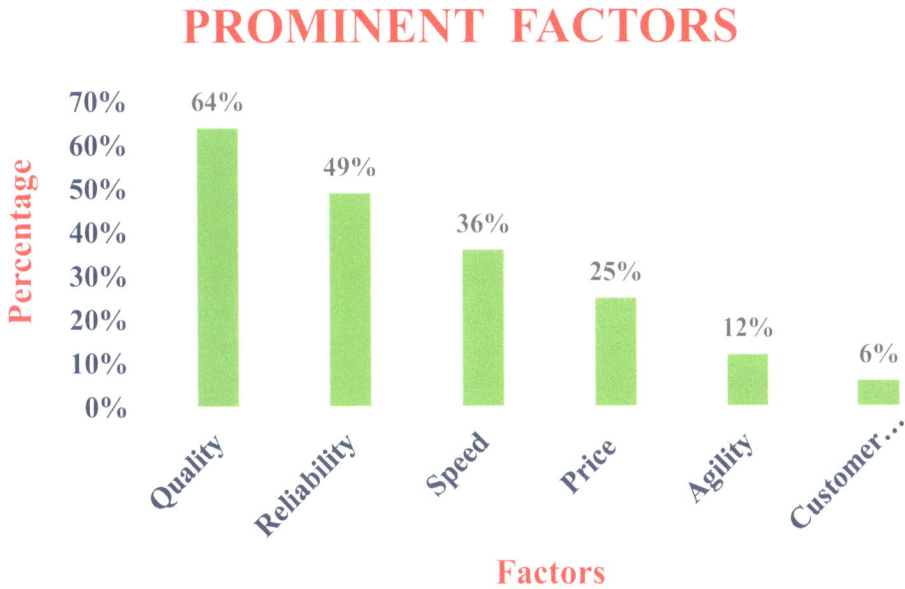

Fig. (2). Prominent factors of a supplier for a customer (Source [44]).

Lessons Learned from COVID-19 for Constructing the Production Process for the Future

Make a plan to adapt to changing circumstances

In this pandemic, many manufacturers realized the hard way that their contingency plans were inadequate. For planning in the forthcoming years, extensive deep research into the supply chain is required including analyzing potentially tier three suppliers for any flaws. Make sure some alternatives are readily available and easily accessible. Include more local vendors in your strategy and develop a plan to operate in the short term to improve cash flow instead of profits, and examine your industry's product portfolio and consumer base to establish priorities.

Demand Volatility can be Managed with On-demand Production

On-demand industrial production could help businesses to handle demand volatility, manage inventory costs, and deliver the exact products at the right time for the optimum overall cost. Manufacturing on demand allows businesses to avoid being tethered to enormous production estimates, allowing them to better navigate volatility in the market. Parts could be manufactured quickly as demand spikes. Since there is no longer an emphasis on manufacturing new products with high minimum order quantities, on-demand procurement could also reduce total inventory costs.

Supply Chains Benefit from Mass Customizations

A mass customization strategy is another technique to manage supply chain interruptions. The demands of today's market are increasingly personalized, t This limited, quick proportion of items is not the same as the production process of the former when mass production was the typical benchmark. Customization is reshaping the way how production should respond, and on-demand manufacturing does have digital capacity and capability to meet mass customization demands.

A Worldwide Network Built on the Backbone of Regional Vendors

Companies can avoid global disturbances by using regional suppliers, especially if those regional suppliers engage regional suppliers as well. Many organizations have discovered the advantages of on-shoring alternatives, reaping the benefits of contract manufacturers who employ digital technologies under their shores to protect their businesses from macroeconomic volatility. At Protolabs, regionalized and on-demand manufacturing is becoming increasingly popular as a replacement for offshoring. The growth of digital manufacturing has made manufacturing to be done remotely, or nearer to the consumption stage and more financially possible.

CONCLUSION

Companies have never faced as many complications as they do now as a result of macro conditions. Industry 4.0 is defined as a set of digital data-driven networked information technology used in the manufacturing sector to facilitate managing the product and equipment life cycle. Industry 4.0 promotes the integration of organizational learning, people, robots, and commodities, and uses an integrated unified environment to visibly manage logistics, production, process, and data flow. For each ability afforded by digital manufacturing, each product leader ought to have an evaluation strategy and a well-stated position. The problems have shown a key reality about supply chain operations that they can't thrive without flexibility and efficiency. COVID-19 has accelerated Industry 4.0 by recognizing that digital manufacturing is still not only a commercial differentiator but also a requirement in the 21st century.

ACKNOWLEDGMENTS

All authors contributed to the study conception and design. Material preparation, data collection and analysis were performed by Hari Priya and Rajeswari. The first draft of the manuscript was written by Hari Priya and Gunavathi. All authors read and approved the final manuscript.

REFERENCES

[1]   B.S. Mohan, and N. Vinod, "COVID-19: An Insight into SARS-CoV2 Pandemic Originated at Wuhan City in Hubei Province of China", *Journal of Infectious Diseases and Epidemiology,* vol. 6, no. 4, pp. 1-8, 2020.
[http://dx.doi.org/10.23937/2474-3658/1510146]

[2]   M.A. Dar, B. Gladysz, and A. Buczacki, "Impact of covid19 on operational activities of manufacturing organizations - a case study and industry 4.0-based survive-stabilise-sustainability (3s) framework", *Ener.,* vol. 14, no. 7, p. 1900, 2021.
[http://dx.doi.org/10.3390/en14071900]

[3]   L.D. Xu, E.L. Xu, and L. Li, "Industry 4.0: state of the art and future trends", *Int. J. Prod. Res.,* vol. 56, no. 8, pp. 2941-2962, 2018.
[http://dx.doi.org/10.1080/00207543.2018.1444806]

[4]   M.S. Kumar, D.R.D. Raut, D.V.S. Narwane, and D.B.E. Narkhede, "Applications of industry 4.0 to overcome the COVID-19 operational challenges", *Diabetes Metab. Syndr.,* vol. 14, no. 5, pp. 1283-1289, 2020.
[http://dx.doi.org/10.1016/j.dsx.2020.07.010] [PMID: 32755822]

[5]   J. Qin, Y. Liu, and R. Grosvenor, "A categorical framework of manufacturing for industry 4.0 and beyond", *Procedia CIRP,* vol. 52, pp. 173-178, 2016.
[http://dx.doi.org/10.1016/j.procir.2016.08.005]

[6]   S. Wang, J. Wan, D. Li, and C. Zhang, "Implementing Smart Factory of Industrie 4.0: An Outlook", *Int. J. Distrib. Sens. Netw.,* vol. 12, no. 1, p. 3159805, 2016.
[http://dx.doi.org/10.1155/2016/3159805]

[7]   M. Ibrahim, "The fourth industrial revolution combatting COVID-19: the role of smart and sustainable cities", *UNDESA / Division for Inclusive Social Development, in collaboration with UNCTAD and ITU.* **2020**. Available at: https://www.un.org/development/desa/dspd/wp-content/uploads/sites/22/2020/09/Maysoun-Ibrahim_4IR-and-SCs-in-the-Time-of-COVID19.pdf (2020).

[8]   A. Rojko, "Industry 4.0 concept: Background and overview", *International Journal of Interactive Mobile Technologies (iJIM),* vol. 11, no. 5, pp. 77-90, 2017.
[http://dx.doi.org/10.3991/ijim.v11i5.7072]

[9]   J. Butt, "A Conceptual Framework to Support Digital Transformation in Manufacturing Using an Integrated Business Process Management Approach", *Designs.* vol. 4, no. 3, Sep 2020.
[http://dx.doi.org/10.3390/designs4030017]

[10]   M. Ghobakhloo, "The future of manufacturing industry: a strategic roadmap toward Industry 4.0", *J. Manuf. Tech. Manag.,* vol. 29, no. 6, pp. 910-936, 2018.
[http://dx.doi.org/10.1108/JMTM-02-2018-0057]

[11]   W. Lidong, and W. Guanghui, "Big Data in Cyber-Physical Systems, Digital Manufacturing and Industry 4.0", *International Journal of Engineering and Manufacturing,* vol. 6, no. 4, pp. 1-8, 2016.
[http://dx.doi.org/10.5815/ijem.2016.04.01]

[12]   A. Ustundag, and E. Cevikcan, *Industry 4.0: Managing The Digital Transformation.* Springer Cham,

2018.
[http://dx.doi.org/10.1007/978-3-319-57870-5]

[13]   M. Javaid, A. Haleem, R. Vaishya, S. Bahl, R. Suman, and A. Vaish, "Industry 4.0 technologies and their applications in fighting COVID-19 pandemic", *Diabetes Metab. Syndr.,* vol. 14, no. 4, pp. 419-422, 2020.
[http://dx.doi.org/10.1016/j.dsx.2020.04.032] [PMID: 32344370]

[14]   R.S. Peres, X. Jia, J. Lee, K. Sun, A.W. Colombo, and J. Barata, "Industrial Artificial Intelligence in Industry 4.0 - Systematic Review, Challenges and Outlook", *IEEE Access,* vol. 8, pp. 220121-220139, 2020.
[http://dx.doi.org/10.1109/ACCESS.2020.3042874]

[15]   J. Lee, H. Davari, J. Singh, and V. Pandhare, "Industrial artificial intelligence for industry 4.0-based manufacturing systems", *Manuf. Lett.,* vol. 18, pp. 20-23, 2018.
[http://dx.doi.org/10.1016/j.mfglet.2018.09.002]

[16]   S.K. Routray, P. Sharmila, A. Javali, A.D. Ghosh, and S. Sarangi, "An Outlook of Narrowband IoT for Industry 4.0", *2020 Second International Conference on Inventive Research in Computing Applications (ICIRCA),* pp. 923-926, 2020.
[http://dx.doi.org/10.1109/ICIRCA48905.2020.9182803]

[17]   S. Aheleroff, X. Xu, Y. Lu, M. Aristizabal, J. Pablo Velásquez, B. Joa, and Y. Valencia, "IoT-enabled smart appliances under industry 4.0: A case study", *Adv. Eng. Inform.,* vol. 43, p. 101043, 2020.
[http://dx.doi.org/10.1016/j.aei.2020.101043]

[18]   Z. You, and L. Feng, "Integration of industry 4.0 related technologies in construction industry: a framework of Cyber-Physical System", *IEEE Access,* vol. 8, pp. 122908-122922, 2020.
[http://dx.doi.org/10.1109/ACCESS.2020.3007206]

[19]   C.T. Yen, Y.C. Liu, C.C. Lin, C.C. Kao, W.B. Wang, and Y.R. Hsu, "Advanced manufacturing solution to industry 4.0 trend through sensing network and cloud computing technologies", *IEEE International Conference on Automation Science and Engineering (CASE),* pp. 1150-1152, 2014.
[http://dx.doi.org/10.1109/CoASE.2014.6899471]

[20]   M. Lezzi, M. Lazoi, and A. Corallo, "Cybersecurity for Industry 4.0 in the current literature: A reference framework", *Comput. Ind.,* vol. 103, pp. 97-110, 2018.
[http://dx.doi.org/10.1016/j.compind.2018.09.004]

[21]   F. De Pace, F. Manuri, and A. Sanna, ""Augmented reality system for operator support in human–robot collaborative assembly"", *CIRP Annals,* vol. 65, no. 1, pp. 61-64, 2016.

[22]   C. Salkin, M. Oner, A. Ustundag, and E. Cevikcan, A conceptual framework for Industry 4.0.*In: Industry 4.0: managing the digital transformation* Springer Charm, 2018, pp. 3-23.
[http://dx.doi.org/10.1007/978-3-319-57870-5_1]

[23]   M. Mohamed, "Challenges and benefits of Industry 4.0: an overview", *International Journal of Supply and Operations Management,* vol. 5, no. 3, pp. 256-265, 2018.

[24]   M.K. Habib, and C. Chimsom, "Industry 4. 0: Sustainability and Design Principles", *20th International Conference on Research and Education in Mechatronics (REM),* pp. 1-8, 2019.
[http://dx.doi.org/10.1109/REM.2019.8744120]

[25]   A. Gorkhali, and L.D. Xu, "Enterprise Application Integration in Industrial Integration: A Literature Review", *Journal of Industrial Integration and Management,* vol. 1, no. 4, p. 1650014, 2016.
[http://dx.doi.org/10.1142/S2424862216500147]

[26]   Y. Lu, "Industry 4.0: A survey on technologies, applications and open research issues", *J. Ind. Inf. Integr.,* vol. 6, pp. 1-10, 2017.
[http://dx.doi.org/10.1016/j.jii.2017.04.005]

[27]   A. Syberfeldt, M. Holm, O. Danielsson, L. Wang, and R.L. Brewster, "Support systems on the industrial shop-floors of the future – operators ' perspective on augmented reality", *Procedia CIRP,*

vol. 44, pp. 108-113, 2016.
[http://dx.doi.org/10.1016/j.procir.2016.02.017]

[28] C.J. Bartodziej, *The Concept Industry 4.0 – An. Empirical Analysis of Technologies and Applications in Production Logistics.* Springer Gabler: Wiesbaden, Germany, 2017.

[29] D. Dikhanbayeva, S. Shaikholla, Z. Suleiman, and A. Turkyilmaz, "Assessment of Industry 4.0 Maturity Models by Design Principles", *Sustainability (Basel),* vol. 12, no. 23, p. 9927, 2020.
[http://dx.doi.org/10.3390/su12239927]

[30] H. Gebauer, B. Edvardsson, and M. Bjurko, "The impact of service orientation in corporate culture on business performance in manufacturing companies", *J. Serv. Manag.,* vol. 21, no. 2, pp. 237-259, 2010.
[http://dx.doi.org/10.1108/09564231011039303]

[31] M. Hermann, T. Pentek, and B. Otto, "Design Principles for Industrie 4 . 0 Scenarios: A Literature Review Working Paper A Literature Review", 2015. . Available at: https://www.researchgate.net/publication/307864150_Design_Principles_for_Industrie_40_Scenarios_A_Literature_Review(2015).

[32] C.G. Machado, M.P. Winroth, and E.H.D. Ribeiro da Silva, "Sustainable manufacturing in Industry 4.0: an emerging research agenda", *Int. J. Prod. Res.,* vol. 58, no. 5, pp. 1462-1484, 2020.
[http://dx.doi.org/10.1080/00207543.2019.1652777]

[33] M.A. Berawi, "The role of industry 4.0 in achieving Sustainable Development Goals", *International Journal of Technology,* vol. 10, no. 4, pp. 644-647, 2019.
[http://dx.doi.org/10.14716/ijtech.v10i4.3341]

[34] B.A. Kadir, and O. Broberg, "Human-centered design of work systems in the transition to industry 4.0", *Appl. Ergon.,* vol. 92, p. 103334, 2021.
[http://dx.doi.org/10.1016/j.apergo.2020.103334] [PMID: 33264676]

[35] V. Chamola, V. Hassija, V. Gupta, and M. Guizani, "A Comprehensive Review of the COVID-19 Pandemic and the Role of IoT, Drones, AI, Blockchain, and 5G in Managing its Impact", *IEEE Access,* vol. 8, pp. 90225-90265, 2020.
[http://dx.doi.org/10.1109/ACCESS.2020.2992341]

[36] P. Wellener, H. Manolian, and S. Laaper, "Distinctive traits of digital frontrunners in manufacturing"", *Report, Deloitte Insights,* 2018.

[37] T. Stock, and G. Seliger, "Opportunities of Sustainable Manufacturing in Industry 4.0", *Procedia CIRP,* vol. 40, pp. 536-541, 2016.
[http://dx.doi.org/10.1016/j.procir.2016.01.129]

[38] P. Gregori, V. Martinez, and J.J. Moyano Fernandez, "Basic Actions To Reduce Dropout Rates In Distance Basic Actions To Reduce Dropout Rates In Distance", *Eval. Program Plann.,* vol. 66, pp. 48-52, 2018.
[http://dx.doi.org/10.1016/j.evalprogplan.2017.10.004] [PMID: 29031190]

[39] S. Agrawal, A. Jamwal, and S. Gupta, "Effect of COVID-19 on the Indian Economy and Supply Chain", *preprints.org.* May. 9, 2020. Available at: https://www.preprints.org/manuscript/202005.0148/v1(2020).

[40] N. Fernandes, "Economic effects of coronavirus outbreak (COVID-19) on the world economy,"", In: *Tech.Report* Full Professor of Finance IESE Business School: Spain, 2020, pp. 0-32.
[http://dx.doi.org/10.2139/ssrn.3557504]

[41] S.U. Kumar, D.T. Kumar, B.P. Christopher, and C.G.P. Doss, "The Rise and Impact of COVID-19 in India", *Front. Med. (Lausanne),* vol. 7, p. 250, 2020.
[http://dx.doi.org/10.3389/fmed.2020.00250] [PMID: 32574338]

[42] N. Panchal, R. Kamal, and K. Orgera, "The implications of COVID-19 for mental health and substance use", *Kaiser family foundation,* vol. 21, pp. 1-16. Apr 2021.

[43]   S.K. Schäfer, M.R. Sopp, C.G. Schanz, M. Staginnus, A.S. Göritz, and T. Michael, "Impact of COVID-19 on public mental health and the buffering effect of a sense of coherence", *Psychother. Psychosom.,* vol. 89, no. 6, pp. 386-392, 2020.
[http://dx.doi.org/10.1159/000510752] [PMID: 32810855]

[44]   "Protolabs explanation of Navigating Supply Chain Disruptions with Digital Manufacturing", 2021. Available at: https://www.protolabs.com/resources/guides-and-trend-reports/product-develop-ent-and-the-supply-chain-how-to-survive-a-pandemic-with-digitalmanufacturing(Accessed on: 1st June 2021).

SUBJECT INDEX

A

Acid, polylactic 37
Acute 28, 30
   lung injury 28
   respiratory distress syndrome (ARDS) 30
AI-based 70, 124, 142
   DL technique 142
   healthcare system 70
   technology 124
AI-enabled 72, 83, 84, 87
   camera 83, 84
   robots 72
   technology 87
AI-led technologies 87
Aluminum alloys 37
Amazon computational cloud service 154
ANN architecture 4
AR-VR technology 83
Artificial intelligence 64, 77, 80
   algorithms 77, 80
   system 64
Atomic migration technique 36
Automated robotic processes 83
Automatic spraying technology 56
Automation, insurance 90

B

Blockchain technology 94
Bluetooth 65, 84
   device 84
   technology 65
Broadcast data 51
Business(s) 2, 105, 106, 113, 118, 119, 168, 169, 172, 173, 178, 182, 183, 185, 187, 189, 190, 193
   activities 2
   commerce 119
   conventions 187
   ecosystems 178
   financial 183

C

Cardiac 87, 88
   arrest 88
   problems 87
Cardiovascular 54, 72
   sleep 54
   stress 54
   disease 72
Chronic 81
   diseases 81
   obstructive pulmonary disease (COPD) 81
Cloud 56, 82
   based AI-IoT systems 82
   computing technologies 56
Computed tomography (CT) 48, 63
Computer vision 58, 146
   systems 58
   technology 146
Conjoint triad technique 156
Convolution neural networks (CNN) 65, 127, 128
CORONA epidemic 190
Coronavirus 1, 2, 3, 23, 26, 27, 28, 45, 49, 54, 55, 56, 63, 65, 66, 67, 97, 99, 100, 101, 102, 103, 104, 107, 108, 114, 116, 119, 123
   acute respiratory syndrome 97
   disease 26, 28, 49, 97, 101, 102, 103, 104, 107, 108, 116, 123
   illness 45
   infections 3, 54, 114, 119
   outbreak 67, 108
   pandemic 4, 114
Corti software 88
Cough-based analysis 133
COVID-19 2, 40, 44, 52, 55, 58, 60, 76, 84, 101, 102, 105, 107, 116, 118, 119, 123, 133, 138, 144, 145, 147, 152, 153, 158
   and cyber incidents 76
   combat 40, 44, 55, 152, 153
   contagion pathogen 123

disease 101, 102, 105, 107, 116, 118, 119
  drug repositioning 123
  infection 58, 133
  risk evaluation 123
  screening 158
  symptom identifications 52
  transmission of 2, 60, 138, 144, 145
  vaccine 147
  virus 84, 116
COVID-19 safety 123, 151
  guidelines 151
  measures 123
Crisis 2, 3, 42, 48, 184, 187, 191
  economic 2
  financial 184
  ventilator 42
Cross-sectional 5, 39
  dependence cooccurrences 5
  imaging 39
CT images 63
Cybercriminals 151
Cybersecurity 69, 77, 168, 174, 175

D

Data normalization techniques 4
Deep neural networks (DNN) 127, 132, 157
Depression 187
Detergent consumption 77
Devices 28, 38, 76, 87, 89, 92, 174, 188
  biomedical 76
  communication 174
  mechanical 28
  microelectromechanical 38
  sensing 188
  skin-attachable 87
  telehealth 92
  telemedical 89
  video 87
Digital 30, 180, 191
  fabrication technology 30
  manufacturing method 191
  transformation technologies 180
Disease 28, 81, 89, 97, 98
  cardiovascular 98
  chronic obstructive pulmonary 81
  chronic respiratory 98
  communicable 89
  heart 81
  infectious 28, 97

Disorders, cardiovascular 81

E

ECG sensors 54
Economical technique 146
Electrocardiograms 80, 87
Electron beam melting (EBM) 34
Electronic health record (EHR) 69, 72, 80, 83, 94, 137
Eminent clustering techniques 126
Enterprise resource planning (ERP) 170

F

Facial recognition technology 61
FDA-sanctioned commercial medications 153
Feedforward neural networks (FNN) 127, 128
Fog computing 50, 51
Forecasting COVID-19 transmission 139

G

Generative adversarial networks (GANs) 132
Global positioning system (GPS) 48, 54, 55, 86, 88
Glycosylated spike protein (GSP) 157

H

Healthcare 61, 70, 80, 85, 86, 185
  networks 61
  providers 70, 80, 85, 86, 185

I

IIoT technology 180
Industrial 175, 180, 181
  internet of things (IIoT) 180, 181
  robotic systems 175
Industries 2, 78, 92
  medical 78, 92
  tourism 2
Infections 26, 27, 28, 49, 52, 53, 55, 97, 100, 108, 109, 112, 124, 133, 134, 136, 137
  lung 28, 49
  pulmonary 26, 27
  technique forecasts 136

Information transparency 172
Intercrossed forecasting method 143
International 62, 153
   federation of robotics (IFR) 62
   healthcare policy 153
Internet 55, 69, 70, 74, 75, 76, 77, 78, 80, 88,
    90, 92, 93, 94, 104, 168, 171, 174, 179,
    180
   of drone things (IoDT) 55, 88
   of medical things (IoMT) 69, 70, 90, 92,
    93, 94
   of service (IoS) 179
   of things in healthcare 80
Internet-of-things 78, 183
   devices 78
IoMT 92
   applications 92
   devices 92
IoT 50, 73, 74
   based healthcare system 73
   enabled healthcare services 73
   established system 50
   powered artificial intelligence 74

L

Legal profession 150
Lockdown circumstances 107, 144
Logistic regression (LR) 125, 126, 132, 134
LOM technology 35
Long short-term memory (LSTMs) 6, 128,
   132
Lung 26, 28, 63
   disease 26
   problems 28, 63

M

Machine(s) 5, 8, 30, 33, 36, 60, 66, 74, 75, 77,
    84, 85, 87, 88, 123, 125, 169, 172, 177,
    178, 183, 190
   industrial automation 190
   learning 5, 60, 66, 75, 77, 84, 85, 87, 88,
    123, 125
   producing emergency respiration 30
Magnetic resonance imaging (MRI) 48, 63
Manufacturing systems 175
Mean absolute percentage error (MAPE) 3, 4

Medical emergency response system (MERS)
   88
Memory 91, 128, 137
  gated 128
  muscle 91
Metal-based hybrids 33
Migration 139, 172
  flexible 172
  techniques 139
ML-based 137, 153, 156
   alignment-free technique 156
   forecasting 137
   method 153
Mobility circumstances 149
Money transfers 151
Monitor, health investigators 64

N

Natural language processing (NLP) 75, 137,
   150
Netflix application 118
Network 73, 74, 77, 109, 110, 113, 114, 128,
    169, 174, 181, 182
  intelligent 169
Neural network(s) 1, 6, 17, 18, 23, 90, 127,
    128, 140, 142, 151
   regression 18, 23
Neurons 4, 6, 127, 142
  artificial 4
  virtual 127

O

Online 147, 151
   education system 151
   health misconceptions 147
Online learning 110, 111, 151
   resource 111
   systems 151
Otolaryngology 38
Oxygen 26, 27, 28, 29, 87, 130, 159
   cylinders 26, 27
   saturation 159
   therapeutics 130

P

Pandemic 2, 26, 27, 45, 48, 49, 58, 59, 60, 61,
    69, 70, 90, 97, 103, 104, 112, 113, 114,
    115, 119, 137, 146, 148, 168, 169, 187
    combat 168
    crisis 146
    dangerous 26
    disease 48
    global 187
    outbreaks 69, 70, 90
Pathogen genomes 133
Peptide connection 157
Periodic vaccinations 186
Photo 26, 146, 147
    polymerization 26
    preprocessing 146
    ultra-resolution 146, 147
Photopolymerization 37
Photosensitive liquid 34
Platforms, fastest digital manufacturing 190
Pneumonia, aspiration 28
Polynomial regression (PR) 126, 143
Population density 138, 139, 141
Population-level activities 149
Porosis 72
PPE and respiration support devices
    transportation 30
Printing technology 26, 31, 32, 33, 37, 38, 39,
    40, 41, 43
    3-Dimensional 33, 39
    additive 37, 38, 39, 40
Proactive disease treatment 81
Proteins 28, 66, 154
    immune 154
Prothrombin activity 132
Pulmonary damage 28

R

Ramifications 149
Random forest regression (RFR) 126
Regression 126
    analysis 126
    technique 126
Remote patient monitoring (RPM) 91, 94
Resources, medical 134
Respiration rate (RR) 48, 53, 55, 56, 87, 126
Respiratory 49, 55, 186

disorder 186
    Sinus arrhythmia (RSA) 55
    syndrome 49
Reverse transcription polymerase chain
    reaction 63, 131
RF classification technique 135
Risk 99, 135, 136
    assessments 99, 136
    factors 135
Robotic(s) 59, 60, 62, 63, 74, 83, 124, 176,
    181
    assistants 83
    system 59
    technology 59
Robots 52, 59, 60, 61, 62, 67, 71, 75, 77, 83,
    173, 175, 181, 183
    automatic 60
    autonomous 173, 175, 181
    industrial 62
Root mean squared 4, 126, 140, 141
    error (RMSE) 4, 126
    logarithmic errors (RMSLE) 140, 141
RT-PCR 133, 158
    approach 133
    method 158

S

SARS-CoV-2 28, 132, 135, 154, 157, 158,
    160
    illness 132
    infection 28, 135
    outbreak 160
    pathogen 157, 158
    protein structure 157
    targeted proteins 154
Selective laser sintering (SLS) 34, 35
Sensor(s) 50, 73, 74, 75, 76, 80, 81, 82, 87,
    88, 124, 136, 137, 159, 172, 173, 178,
    183
    acoustic 50
    facial recognition 124
    mobile 159
    networks 82
Sequences 131, 155, 156
    nucleotide 131
    viral genomic 156
    virus-antibody 155
Service integration systems 171
Siamese neural network (SNN) 157

Skills 58, 110, 111
  decision-making 110
Sleep disturbances 87
Sliding window method 143
Smart 69, 77, 78, 87, 175
    contact lenses 87
    laundry machines 77
    manufacturing production process 175
    medical sensors and Internet-of-things
        devices 78
    wearables 69, 87
Social 2, 27, 104, 117, 118, 145
    communication 104
    density 145
    distancing rules 2, 27, 117, 118
Social media 97, 99, 100, 101, 102, 104, 106,
    107, 108, 109, 111, 112, 113, 114, 116,
    117, 118
    applications 117
    demeanor 116
    marketing 113
    networks 97, 99, 108, 111
Socioeconomic information 144
Software, descriptive statistical 4
Speech alarms, real-time 146
Spikes, repetitive 140
Sporting events 151
Stereolithography 36
Stress hormone 54
Support 27, 48, 66, 125, 126, 132, 134, 136,
    138
    healthcare workers 27
    vector machine (SVM) 48, 66, 125, 132,
        134, 136, 138
    vector regression (SVR) 126
Surgery 38, 59, 71, 72
  lung 38
  maxillofacial 38
  orthopaedic 38
  plastic 38
  robotic 59, 72
Sustainable production 180
Synthetic immunoglobulins 155

T

Technologies 64, 74, 99, 190
  computer-mediated 99
  infrared 64
  robust 74

    smart 190
Telemedicine facilities 73
Therapeutic pathway 136
Thermal imaging 55
Throat, sore 49

U

Unmanned aircraft vehicles (UAVs) 55, 88

V

Vaccines 26, 27, 29, 49, 66, 67, 84, 89, 152,
    155, 187
    preventive 27
    tuberculosis 155
Vaxign reversal vaccinology technique 155
Ventilator 40, 130
    machines 40
    systems 130
Viral 54, 156
    infections 54
    infestations 156
Virtualized embedded system 181
Virus 1, 2, 3, 23, 26, 27, 63, 64, 97, 98, 124,
    133, 134, 144, 148, 184, 186
    disease-causing 148
    mutates 124
Visual information 128
Voice recordings 136

W

Wald test 5
Waste 182
    production 182
    reduction 182
Wearable(s) 80, 91
    consumer health 91
    fitness devices 80
Wireless communication 183

www.ingramcontent.com/pod-product-compliance
Lightning Source LLC
Chambersburg PA
CBHW050841220326
41598CB00006B/430